W9-BUB-365

LIVING WITH SCOLIOSIS

LIVING WITH SCOLIOSIS

by L. E. Carmichael

Content Consultant

William K. Accousti, MD, Associate Professor of Orthopaedic Surgery—Louisiana State University Health Sciences Center, Orthopaedic Surgeon—Children's Hospital New Orleans

LIVING WITH HEALTH CHALLENGES

CREDITS

Published by ABDO Publishing Company, PO Box 398166, Minneapolis, MN 55439. Copyright © 2014 by Abdo Consulting Group, Inc. International copyrights reserved in all countries. No part of this book may be reproduced in any form without written permission from the publisher. The Essential Library™ is a trademark and logo of ABDO Publishing Company.

Printed in the United States of America,
North Mankato, Minnesota
092013
012014

♻ THIS BOOK CONTAINS AT LEAST 10% RECYCLED MATERIALS.

Editor: Jenna Gleisner
Series Designer: Becky Daum

Photo credits: George Doyle/Thinkstock, cover, 3; Jupiterimages/Thinkstock, 8; Thinkstock, 11, 12, 80; Fuse/Thinkstock, 18, 26, 68; Shutterstock Images, 21, 25, 66; Ingram Publishing/Thinkstock, 28; AJPhoto/Custom Medical, 31; Wavebreak Media/Thinkstock, 33; Digital Vision/Thinkstock, 38; Thinkstock, 42, 44, 48, 55, 56, 58, 71, 88, 94; Francis Wong Chee Yen/Shutterstock Images, 63; Apples Eyes Studio/Shutterstock Images, 73; Monkey Business Images/iStockphoto, 75; Shutterstock Images, 83; Chris Clinton/Thinkstock, 96

Library of Congress Control Number: 2013945896

Cataloging-in-Publication Data

Carmichael, L. E.
 Living with scoliosis / L. E. Carmichael.
  p. cm. -- (Living with health challenges)
Includes bibliographical references and index.
ISBN 978-1-62403-247-9
1. Scoliosis--Juvenile literature. 2. Spine--Abnormalities--Juvenile literature.   I. Title.
616.7--dc23

2013945896

CONTENTS

EXPERT ADVICE

I attended medical school at Georgetown University in Washington, DC, and after finishing my orthopaedic surgery residency, I came to Children's Hospital in New Orleans for an additional year of specialty training in pediatric orthopaedic and scoliosis surgery. Afterward, I stayed on staff at the Children's Hospital and became an associate professor of orthopaedic surgery at Louisiana State University Health Sciences Center.

As a child, I was noticed to have a spinal curvature during a school screening. It turned out to be mild scoliosis, but I remember feeling something was seriously wrong with me. As time went on and over the many years I have treated patients with similar spinal issues, I have come to realize it is nothing to worry about.

I have performed all aspects of pediatric spinal deformity surgery in children of all ages, but I perform the most surgeries on teenagers with scoliosis. After treating hundreds of children and teenagers with spinal deformities and scoliosis, I have come to appreciate the fears and apprehension that go along with the diagnosis, but I also see how well patients do after treatment.

My advice to teens with scoliosis is this: stay fit and flexible through regular exercise, wear your brace the way your doctor instructs if you have been prescribed a brace, and realize scoliosis surgery, if needed, is not a disabling but rather an enabling procedure. Lastly, if you are diagnosed with scoliosis, remember you are not alone. Scoliosis is a frequent and somewhat common condition. Scoliosis surgery, although complex and serious, is one of the safest and most reliable procedures we perform in pediatric orthopaedics. The majority of patients who need corrective spinal fusion operations will be able to return to all of life's typical activities. So do not panic if your doctor tells you and your family your spine curvature requires surgery.

— William K. Accousti, MD, Associate Professor of Orthopaedic Surgery at Louisiana State University Health Sciences Center and Orthopaedic Surgeon at Children's Hospital New Orleans

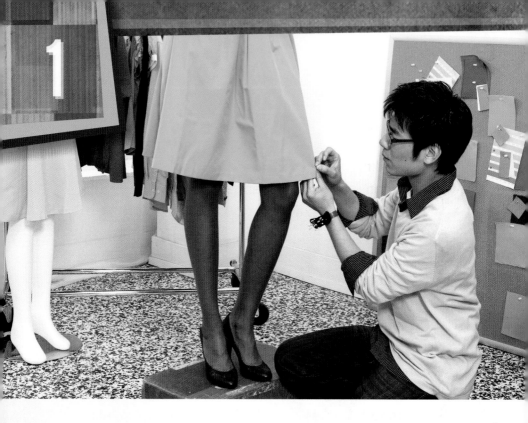

GOING SIDEWAYS

"That dress is so amazing on you," Jess said. "Justin's gonna lose it!"

Lauren couldn't stop staring at herself in the three-way mirrors. Jess was right—the dress was made for her. Except for the length, of course, which was why she was

As milder cases of scoliosis often do not cause pain, you may not know you have scoliosis until clothing fits a different way.

standing in heels, waiting to be measured for alterations. She'd never had a date for a school dance before, and she wanted everything to be perfect.

The tailor appeared with a tape measure in hand and a pincushion strapped to his wrist. Lauren chatted to Jess about transportation plans for the dance while the man knelt in front of her, folding up the dress's hem. He folded and refolded and measured over and over again, as if the math just didn't add up. "Something wrong?" Lauren asked, rolling her eyes at Jess.

The tailor didn't reply for a moment, just got up and circled behind her. In the mirror, Lauren saw him staring at her shoulder blades, visible over the dress's low back. She just started to feel creeped out when he said, "Oh, that explains it. You have scoliosis."

"No, I don't," Lauren replied automatically.

"What's scoliosis?" Jess asked.

"Her spine is curved." The tailor drew a wavy line in the air and met Lauren's gaze in the glass. "It's no problem," he said with a smile. "I'll just hem it on an angle, and it will look straight to the eye."

He picked up his tape measure and went back to work. Jess shrugged and whipped out her cell phone to answer a text. Lauren stared at her reflection again, but all she saw was that wavy line. How could something be wrong with her and she never even knew it?

A CLOSE LOOK AT YOUR SPINE

You probably don't spend much time thinking about your spine, but it's a complex and crucial part of your anatomy. It supports your weight against the forces of gravity, allowing you to walk upright. It gives you the flexibility to bend over when you drop your pencil in class. And it protects your spinal cord—the nerve highway connecting your brain to the rest of your body. The spine is composed of a series of bones called vertebrae, which are separated by rubbery round discs that provide cushioning and shock absorption. Muscles and ligaments connect the vertebrae, keeping them aligned one on top of the next.

Each vertebra has a donut-shaped body, and their stacked holes create a channel for the spinal cord. Vertebrae also have three bony protrusions called processes. The spinous processes cause the bumps you feel when you run a finger down your back; two transverse processes extend from the sides of each vertebrae. In the chest, transverse processes connect the vertebrae to the ribs.

Depending on your age, you may have anywhere from 26 to 32 vertebrae. That's

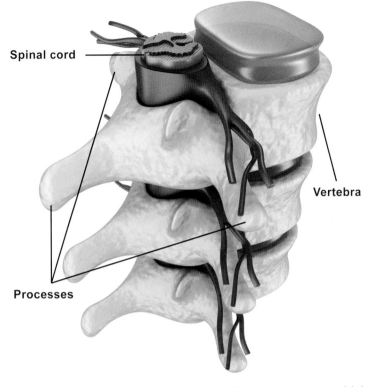

Spinal cord

Vertebra

Processes

Each vertebra has three processes, which somewhat resemble the arms on a starfish.

because the six vertebrae in your pelvis fuse together as you grow. The remaining vertebrae are classified according to location and function. The cervical vertebrae are found in your neck. They are known as C1 through C7. C1 connects your skull to your spine and is sometimes called atlas, after the Greek myth of the titan who holds the weight of the world on his back. The thoracic vertebrae are located in your chest. T1 through T12 attach to your ribs. Lastly, the lumbar vertebrae run from your lower back to your pelvis. L1 through L5 are both the largest

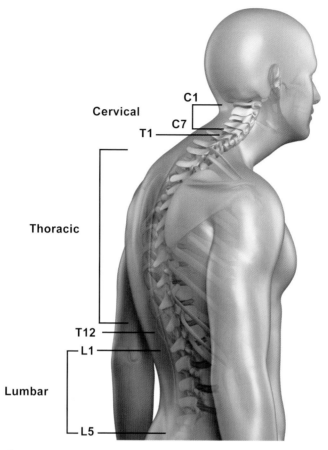

C1

Cervical

C7

T1

Thoracic

T12

L1

Lumbar

L5

The front-to-back S-shaped curves of a healthy spine are normal and necessary for standing upright.

vertebrae and those most responsible for flexibility.

CURVES AND TWISTS

When seen from the side, a healthy spine is S-shaped, curving backward through the chest and forward in the lower back. Viewed from behind, however, vertebrae should form a straight line down the center of the body. If your spine moves from left to right in one or more curves, you might have scoliosis. From an ancient Greek word meaning "crooked," scoliosis is not a disease but a symptom. It can be caused by a number of conditions and has been recognized for more than 2,000 years.

Curve patterns vary among patients, but four types are most common:

- *Thoracic*—these curves are the most common form of scoliosis. These C-shaped curves usually start between T4 and T6 and end between T11 and L1.

- *Thoracolumbar*—these curves are also C-shaped. They involve vertebrae from T4 to as low as L4. They can shift the spine to the left or the right.

- *Lumbar*—these curves form a C-shaped pattern that affects vertebrae between T11 and L5 and points to the left 70 percent of the time.[1]

- *Double major*—these S-shaped curves are the most common type of scoliosis. Double majors include thoracic curves and lumbar curves with opposite orientations.

Depending on the severity, scoliosis curves can cause the body to look unbalanced. Your waist, hips, or shoulders may appear uneven, or one shoulder blade might seem more prominent. For females, asymmetry in the chest can also cause one breast to appear larger than the other.

In addition to shifting away from the center of the body, vertebrae involved in scoliosis often rotate so their backward-facing spinous processes turn to the side instead. If rotation affects the thoracic vertebrae, it causes the ribs to compress, spread, and shift out of normal alignment. The result is a deformity called rib hump.

A MYSTERIOUS DISORDER

Because mild to moderate cases of scoliosis do not cause pain or limit physical activity, many people have no idea they're affected. The Scoliosis Research Society estimates approximately 10 percent of teens have some form of lateral curve.[2] However, roughly only 10 percent of affected teens experience symptoms or complications severe enough to require medical treatment.[3]

KYPHOSIS

The normal, backward curve of the chest vertebrae is called kyphosis. Hyperkyphosis, also known as roundback or hunchback, occurs when this curve is unusually deep. Scheuermann's kyphosis is the most common type. It's caused by wedge-shaped deformations of the vertebrae, and it usually affects boys between the ages of 12 and 15 years.[4]

It's also possible to develop abnormal curves in the lower back. An unusually deep curve causes what is called swayback, while a shallow curve causes flatback. All of these conditions can affect posture or cause pain.

Many believe scoliosis to be a woman's condition, as it is most often detected in girls. In truth, the disorder affects girls and boys equally. However, curves in girls are ten times more likely to get worse, and girls are five times more likely to need medical care.[5] Scientists don't know why this gender bias exists, but it's something female patients need to keep in mind.

STRUCTURE OR FUNCTION?

Structural scoliosis is a growth disorder that alters the skeletal framework of the body. Functional scoliosis is quite different. In this condition, a patient's spine appears curved when standing but straightens out when bending or lying down. Functional scoliosis can be caused by muscle spasms, uneven muscle development, poor posture, injury, or differences in leg length. Unlike the structural form, functional scoliosis has no permanent effect on the spine and can be cured by treating the underlying condition.

CATCHING THE CURVE

Many scoliosis curves go undetected until they are quite severe. This is partially because some types of curves don't cause much deformity. It's also because teens with noticeable asymmetry may be embarrassed by it and use clothing or behaviors to disguise the shape of their bodies.

Successful treatment depends on catching the curve early. Signs you may have scoliosis

SCHOOL SCREENING

Until recently, approximately 30 US states had mandatory school screening programs for scoliosis.[6] The goal was to catch spinal deformities early so treatment could begin before health complications developed. These programs were often too sensitive. Many kids were sent to specialists with curves so small they would never need medical attention. As a result, most states have canceled their screening programs. The incidence of scoliosis hasn't changed, though, and in some patients, it develops very quickly. Ask your doctor to test you at every routine checkup just to be safe.

include comments from adults who keep telling you to stand up straight, top or bra straps that always slide off one shoulder, and skirts or dresses that look as if they're hemmed crooked. If you've noticed these things, use a full-length mirror to look for asymmetry in your hips, waist, shoulders, or shoulder blades. It is possible for scoliosis to develop suddenly, so check yourself periodically and ask your doctor about anything unusual.

ASK YOURSELF THIS

- *Why do you think a stranger was the first to notice something unusual about Lauren's spine?*

- *Do you ever have trouble with clothes that don't hang properly?*

- *Have you noticed asymmetry in a friend's torso while swimming or at the beach?*

- *What medical complications would you expect to arise from a misaligned or rotated spine?*

- *Did your elementary school or junior high have a scoliosis screening program? If you or a classmate were referred to specialists, what was the outcome?*

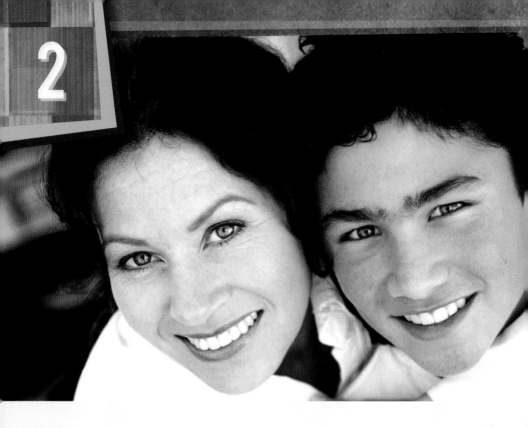

OF NO KNOWN ORIGIN

Nick stood in his swim trunks in the living room, trying not to shiver. February was not exactly bathing suit season, but his mom insisted. It had been six months since she checked his back, and he couldn't put her off any longer. Nick's mom never talked about her

*While researchers are unsure of the cause of
scoliosis, it is known that genes can play a role.*

scoliosis, but he knew it bothered her a lot. Why
else would she keep putting him through this?

"Can we make this quick, Mom?" he called.
"I'm going to miss the movie."

"Sorry, honey," she said, coming in from the
hall. "I'll be quick." She stood behind him, pulling
his shoulders back. Nick tried not to fidget as
her hands moved over his back, his ribs, and
his hips. She put her palms flat on his shoulder
blades. It seemed as if this was taking longer
than usual.

"Nick, can you bend over?" his mom asked,
and her voice sounded a little weird. He sighed
and reached for his toes, a bit surprised when
he couldn't quite touch them. Starting at the
ticklish spot on his neck, she ran a finger down
the bumps of his spine. But instead of plotting a
straight path, he felt her trace a curve. "Oh, no,"
she whispered.

Nick stood up straight and turned around,
stunned to see his mom crying. She pulled him
into her arms, and he hugged her awkwardly as
she sobbed. The only words he could make out
were "I'm sorry."

ADOLESCENT IDIOPATHIC SCOLIOSIS

If you've just been diagnosed with scoliosis, you're probably wondering if there's something you did or didn't do to cause the condition. The answer is no. Slouching and certain sports do not cause scoliosis. Unfortunately, despite decades of intensive research, scientists still don't know what does. Between 80 and 85 percent of the time, scoliosis is idiopathic, meaning the origin is not known.[1] Adolescent idiopathic scoliosis (AIS), which develops between ages 10 and 16, is the most common type. Approximately 2 to 4 percent of teens are affected.[2]

PRESENT FROM BIRTH

In rare cases, vertebrae form incorrectly during the first six weeks of fetal development. These defects cause congenital scoliosis, meaning it is present from birth. The cause is unknown, but if pregnant mice are exposed to certain chemicals, their pups are sometimes affected. A breed of dog called the King Charles spaniel can also develop congenital scoliosis, so it's likely there is a genetic link as well.

Children with congenital scoliosis may have vertebrae that are abnormally connected or shaped as triangles instead of rectangles. Conditions that cause these bone malformations can also affect organs forming at the same phase of fetal development. As a result, patients have a 25 percent chance of developing kidney problems and a 10 percent chance of experiencing heart defects.[3]

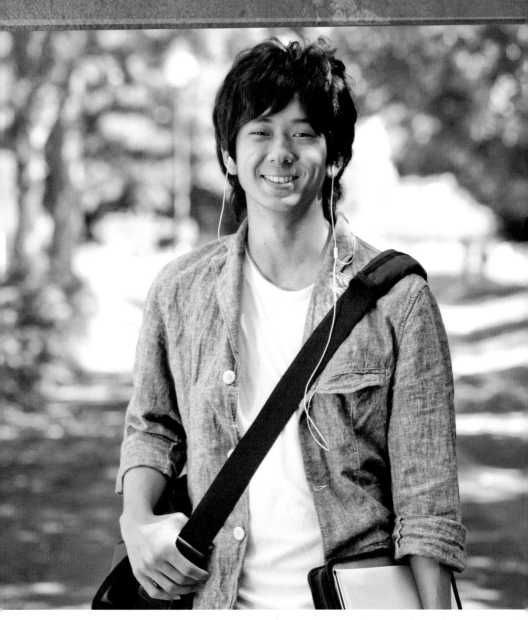

Contrary to myth, carrying a heavy backpack does not cause scoliosis.

KEEPING IT IN THE FAMILY

Animal research is a powerful tool for studying human disease, and since the 1950s, scientists have modeled scoliosis in everything from

INFANTILE IDIOPATHIC SCOLIOSIS

Though unusual, some children develop scoliosis before age three. Because the reason is unknown, this early-onset form is called infantile idiopathic scoliosis (IIS). IIS usually appears as a left thoracic curve. It is more common in European children than in the United States, and it affects boys more often than girls. In most cases, kids with IIS are perfectly healthy except for their curve.

frogs to chickens to goats. This research supports two major theories about AIS. Some scientists believe defective nerves or back muscles place abnormal stress on the spine, pulling it out of position. Experiments with frogs suggest nerves in the ear, which influence balance, movement, and posture, may also be involved.

The second theory is that spines with scoliosis are similar to badly built architectural columns—if they can't support body weight against gravity, they deform. Rats develop scoliosis only when their spines are held perpendicular to the ground, suggesting the human habit of walking upright is in itself a risk factor for AIS.

The only fact we know for sure is genes are involved in AIS. Approximately 30 percent of patients come from families with a history of scoliosis.[4] Your risk also increases when a brother or sister is affected, even if your parents aren't.

GENE HUNTING

Many genes that affect growth and development in humans play a similar role in animals. Because small mammals and fish are easy to breed and study in a lab, scientists can identify genes linked to scoliosis in animals. Scientists can then test to see whether these genes are also found in human scoliosis patients. Candidate genes that affect connective tissue, bone formation, brain chemistry, puberty, and growth have all been tested, but so far, no clear cause of human AIS has been found using this method.

JUVENILE IDIOPATHIC SCOLIOSIS

Juvenile idiopathic scoliosis (JIS) is diagnosed in children between the ages of four and ten. At the younger end of the spectrum, boys with left curves are most common. Older patients are most often girls with curves that shift right.

Twenty percent of kids with severe forms of JIS have an underlying medical condition.[5] One of these is the Chiari malformation, in which the lower part of the brain droops into the spinal column. Chiari malformations also cause scoliosis in King Charles spaniels. Brain surgery to repair this problem may also cure the scoliosis. Patients whose JIS is truly idiopathic, however, have a long road ahead. Their curves progressively worsen and may cause serious health complications.

Genetic technology is always improving, and many scientists are using a new strategy to hunt scoliosis genes. First, they look for DNA markers that are more common in affected families than in the general population. Next, they figure out what those genes do and whether it's logical their functions would be involved in the condition.

SCOLIOSIS AS A SYMPTOM

Doctors used to believe AIS was caused by mild infections of the polio virus. We now know this is incorrect, but scoliosis is a symptom of several other conditions affecting nerves and muscles. These include Duchenne muscular dystrophy, a genetic disorder causing muscle weakness; neurofibromatosis, in which tumors form along the nerves; and spinal cord injuries that lead to paralysis.

These types of scoliosis worsen over time, and, lung, kidney, and digestive problems can also be caused by the original condition.

A COMPLICATED, CONFUSING CONDITION

Identifying the source of AIS has been challenging for two main reasons. One is that scoliosis travels differently through different families. It may be passed from one affected parent to his or her child or passed strictly from mother to son. Sometimes, children of parents with scoliosis are completely healthy. And sometimes,

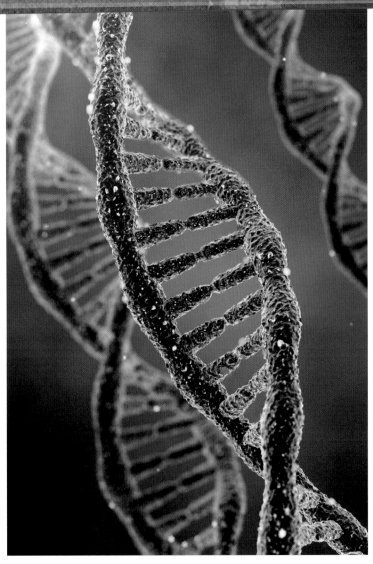

Some nervous system genes have been linked to scoliosis.

scoliosis pops in and out of family trees without any apparent pattern whatsoever. These conflicting results mean there is no single scoliosis gene. Instead, many different genes contribute to the development of AIS.

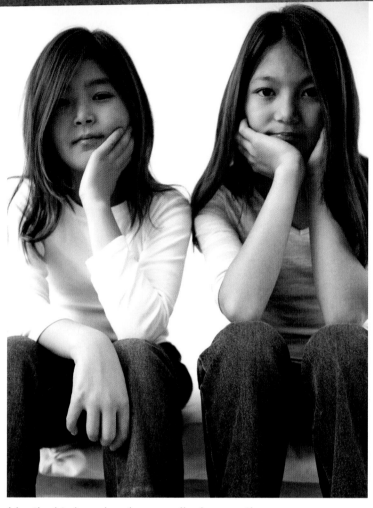

Identical twins who share scoliosis sometimes develop different curve patterns.

Second, the chance that identical twins will both have scoliosis is only 73 percent.[6] This suggests that genes and unknown environmental factors combine to produce scoliosis. Despite these difficulties, many scientists remain optimistic. As research methods continue to improve, we get closer to finding the real causes of idiopathic scoliosis.

ASK YOURSELF THIS

- *Why do you think Nick's mom apologized when she discovered his scoliosis?*

- *Are there any cases of scoliosis in your family? If so, does your doctor know you're at an increased risk?*

- *Does it surprise you that after 2,000 years the cause of scoliosis is still largely unknown?*

- *How do you feel about the use of animals in scoliosis research? What advantages and disadvantages do you see in this approach?*

ADULT-ONSET SCOLIOSIS

Sometimes, adults who had straight spines as teenagers develop scoliosis later in life. Adult scoliosis often starts with arthritis, which causes a breakdown of the discs between the vertebrae. In women, menopause and osteoporosis are also linked to onset of adult scoliosis.

As well as curves and rib humps, patients with adult scoliosis may have problems maintaining upright posture. Pain is also much more common for adult patients than for teens. It can be caused by overworked muscles or by pressure shrinking discs might be placing on nerves in the spine.

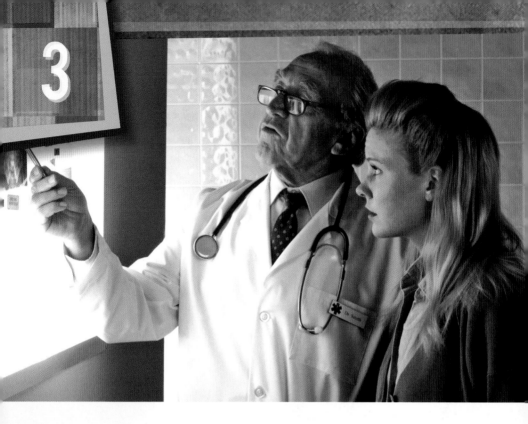

EXAMS AND X-RAYS

E ve had never been happier to be fully
dressed.

The idea people might be looking at
her body had always made her uncomfortable—
even more so since puberty kicked in. Unlike
most girls her age, she wore long sleeves and

Looking at X-rays of your scoliosis for the first time can be shocking and difficult to accept.

hated bathing suits. The worst day of her life had been when she forgot to lock the bathroom door and her dad walked in while she was changing.

Until today.

Dad had always had a tendency to overreact, but Eve had no idea why he thought her weird little waist dent required a trip to the doctor. Especially a doctor who made her walk around in her underwear while he squinted at her and took photographs. She'd never felt so vulnerable and humiliated. At least she got to wear a gown for the X-rays, even if it had been impossible to keep it from gaping open in the back.

The doctor walked in with the X-rays. Eve tugged at her collar, crossing her arms over her chest while the doctor clipped the films to a screen on the wall. When he hit the lights, she couldn't stop herself from blurting, "Those aren't mine."

He gave her a sympathetic smile. "I'm afraid they are, Eve." With a pencil, he pointed to the curves on the image, one balanced over the other. "This S-pattern is the reason you didn't notice it sooner—your curves are pretty evenly matched. But they are severe enough for us to discuss treatment."

The doctor started telling her parents about the options, but Eve wasn't listening. She was mesmerized by the image of that twisted spine. It couldn't be hers. There had to be some kind of mistake.

SPECIAL DOCTORS FOR SPECIAL CIRCUMSTANCES

Because AIS is relatively rare, family doctors might never have seen a case or might not be familiar with the latest research. If you suspect you're affected, you'll need to visit an orthopedic specialist—a bone doctor. The specialist's first goal is figuring out if you have scoliosis, and if so, what type. He or she will ask about your family history and any symptoms that might point to an underlying cause. If you're in pain, for example, your scoliosis may be due to a cracked vertebra or a disc bulging between the bones. Before a diagnosis can be

FUSED BONES

As you grow, bones called the iliac apophysis first form, then migrate toward the top of each hip. By the time your body is completely mature, these bones will have fused with your pelvis. Doctors use the Risser scale to describe which step in this process your bones have reached. At Risser 0, the iliac apophysis has not yet formed; by Risser 5, fusion is complete. The chance your scoliosis will progress decreases after Risser 3.

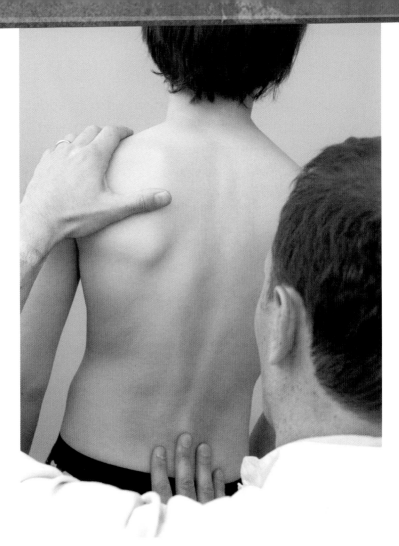

Because scoliosis alters your spine in all three dimensions, the specialist will study your shape from the back, the front, and the side.

made, however, the specialist must also conduct a complete exam.

THE PHYSICAL EXAM

Most teens find the idea of undressing in front of others pretty horrifying. But it's the only way the doctor can get a good look at your bones. It's important to know what to expect. You'll be asked to strip down to your underwear. Female patients should be prepared to remove their bras in case the doctor needs to check their breasts. If you have long hair, pin it up so it doesn't hide your neck and shoulders. During the exam, your doctor will ask you to let your arms hang loosely and look straight ahead.

After looking for asymmetry, your doctor may check your reflexes or ask you to walk around. This helps reveal any muscle or nerve problems and whether your legs are the same length. Finally, the specialist will perform an

THE APEX AND THE ANGLE

Curve pattern is determined by the location of the apex vertebra—the one farthest from the center of the body—and convexity. In a right thoracic curve, for example, the apex vertebrae is on the right side of the chest. If a patient is lying on the left side, the curve would look similar to a mountain with the apex vertebrae at its peak.

The Cobb angle measures the relative height of the mountain—the severity of the curve. To calculate the Cobb angle, doctors use X-rays to identify the topmost and bottommost vertebrae involved. They draw a straight line off the edge of each endpoint, add perpendicular lines to those, and use a protractor to measure the angle of intersection.

The measurements of one patient's Cobb angle can vary by up to 5 degrees, depending on the endpoints chosen and who does the calculation. Consistency across measurements helps distinguish between human error and real changes in the severity of a curve.

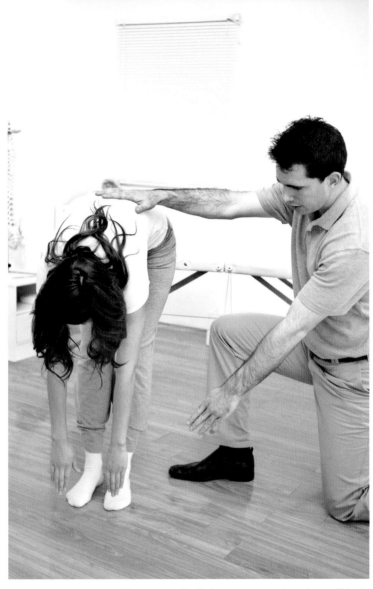

Even small rib humps are clearly visible in the Adams Forward Bend Test position.

Adams Forward Bend Test. If your vertebrae have rotated, causing a rib hump, bending makes its severity easier to measure.

EXPOSING THE BONES

If your doctor finds abnormalities during the physical exam, spinal X-rays are the next step. Depending on your situation, X-rays may be taken from the front, back, or side. You may be asked to stand up straight or lie down. If your doctor needs to check your flexibility, you'll bend away from your curve while an image is taken. These bending X-rays show how much your curve straightens out when you stretch. In all cases, you'll be given lead shields to protect you from the radiation. X-rays reveal the shape of your curve, its location, and its direction. They're also used to calculate your Cobb angle—the severity of your curve as measured in degrees. If your angle is greater than ten degrees, you have scoliosis.

Before he or she can recommend a treatment, though, your doctor needs to know

ADAMS FORWARD BEND TEST

The Adams Forward Bend Test for scoliosis is easy and painless:

- Stand with your feet together and knees straight.
- Clasp your hands or press your palms together.
- Bend forward from the waist, letting your head hang down.
- If your doctor finds a rib hump, he or she will use a scoliometer to measure its slope. This simple device rests on your back and works similarly to a carpenter's level. A tilt of seven or more degrees is a sign you'll need an X-ray.

whether you've finished growing. X-rays of your hip or wrist are the best way to tell. Similar to the vertebrae in your pelvis, which gradually fuse as you age, bones in these areas change predictably during growth. They're a more accurate measure of your body's maturity than your age in years.

WHAT COMES NEXT

The first glimpse of X-rays of your curved spine can be shocking. More than 50 percent of patients deny their diagnosis at first.[1] Guilt, grief, anger, and panic are also common reactions to the news.

The first thing you need to know is most cases of scoliosis require no treatment and will have very little effect on your life. However, if your curve is at risk of progressing you'll need to decide how to proceed. The recommended treatment for AIS varies with severity.

If your curve is less than 20 degrees at diagnosis, your doctor will recommend observation. You'll have periodic X-rays to check your spine, but nothing needs to be done unless the curve gets worse. If your curve is between 20 and 40 degrees and you're still growing, your doctor will probably suggest you wear an orthotic to prevent your curve from worsening. If your curve is more than 50 degrees, you

THERE'S AN APP FOR THAT

Doctors have tested smartphone apps that measure rib hump and Cobb angle. They found no significant differences between the accuracy of these apps, traditional scoliometer readings, and manual calculations of Cobb angles.[2] Because iPhones are popular and convenient, they might become common tools for diagnosing scoliosis in the future.

are a candidate for spinal fusion surgery. Fusion prevents progression and usually improves the curves you already have.

When considering your options, remember scoliosis is not an emergency. Take the time to understand the pros and cons of each treatment before making a decision. And if you feel isolated or alone, talk to other scoliosis patients who know exactly what you're going through. Your specialist can put you in touch with teens in similar situations.

ASK YOURSELF THIS

- *Why do you think Eve had such a hard time accepting her diagnosis?*

- *What preparations would make your first visit to a specialist less stressful?*

- *How would a diagnosis of AIS make you feel? How would it complicate your life?*

- *If you have already been diagnosed with AIS, how did you react when you saw your X-rays?*

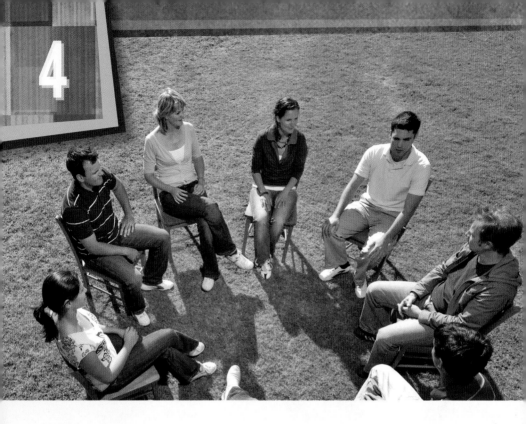

THE PROBLEM OF PROGRESSION

Trey's car came to a stop, and Abby grabbed her stuff. "Let me and the others know what the doctor says," Trey insisted, squeezing her hand. Abby and Trey had been in the same scoliosis support group for almost a year now, and she was glad he understood her scoliosis.

"I will," Abby replied. "See you later!"

She headed up the street to her house, still smiling. Her orthotist was supposed to call today, and she almost skipped her support group meeting to stay home and wait, but she was glad she went. Talking to people who have dreaded the same call calmed her down, and she was ready to hear the news now, either way.

Abby's school friends had no idea she had scoliosis. She just couldn't handle their worry and their questions—she didn't want them to treat her differently, especially when she may never need treatment. It was bad enough her parents had gone into helicopter mode, swirling around her as if their love and concern had the power to keep her curve from progressing. She didn't know how she could have survived the past year without her support group, but she was sure they would be there for her, no matter what happened next.

Abby climbed the porch steps and twisted the knob. The door was barely open when her dad pulled her into a huge bear hug.

"You beat it, kiddo!" he shouted, swinging her around in the air. Abby staggered a bit when he put her down, but her mom was there

SCOLISCORE— PROGRESSION IS IN THE GENES

Between 2009 and 2012, more than 5,000 scoliosis patients were screened with scoliScore, a genetic test measuring risk of progression.[1] Using DNA samples from patients' saliva, scoliScore examines 53 different genes. The test's developers claim it is 99 percent accurate at identifying low risk patients. That increased certainty reduces both a patient's fears and the number of X-rays performed during observation.

to steady her, a firm grasp on her forearms.

"Risser 5, Cobb 22," Mom said, tears shining in her eyes. "It's over."

Abby took a deep breath—the first one she'd had since her diagnosis. She couldn't wait to tell Trey the good news.

WHY DO CURVES GET WORSE?

While we don't know how scoliosis starts, human and animal studies suggest progression happens because of a vicious cycle of uneven bone growth. According to this model, the initial curve distributes weight unevenly on the vertebrae. Increased pressure on the inside of the curve slows growth, while decreased pressure on the outside speeds up growth. As a result, the vertebrae become wedge-shaped rather than rectangular. Wedging worsens the unbalanced pressure, leading to further progression.

PROGRESSION LEADS TO PROBLEMS

Your diagnosis might make you feel helpless and overwhelmed or tempt you to ignore the problem in hopes it will go away. Or maybe you're happy with the way you look and believe you'll be one of the lucky patients whose curves stabilize or correct themselves spontaneously. Although these reactions are completely understandable, ignoring progression may compromise your health and happiness in the long run.

Only 2 to 4 percent of all teens with AIS reach 45 degrees or higher.[2] At this level, there are potential complications. Above 40 degrees, asymmetry or rib humps become more obvious, and poor body image may affect social relationships and self-esteem, potentially leading to risk-taking behaviors, such as abusing illegal substances. You could also have posture problems, leading to pain. If your head is not centered over your pelvis, your muscles

CHECKING IN

Depending on your risk factors, you'll visit your specialist every four to six months. At each visit, your specialist will take scoliometer readings or X-rays to look for progression. Between appointments, you can also monitor yourself. Take photographs to track any changes in your appearance. Observation continues until skeletal maturity, when your risk decreases. After this, you won't need another appointment unless something changes.

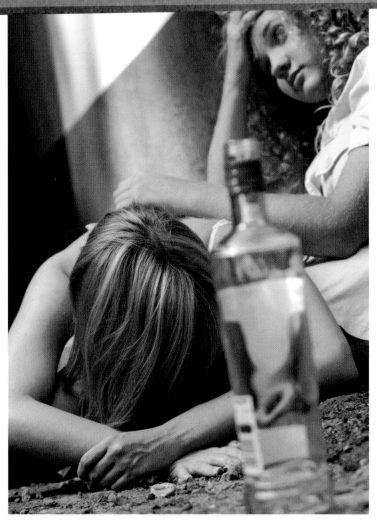

In teens with scoliosis, poor body image has been linked to increased alcohol abuse and suicidal thoughts.

have to work harder to hold you upright, causing fatigue and soreness.

Arthritis, a swelling of the joints, results when tilted vertebrae exert unusual forces on the discs between them, and patients as young as 15 can be affected. In rare cases, misaligned vertebrae pinch the nerves leaving the spinal column. This causes pain, numbness, weakness, or tingling running down the legs. Unfortunately, the usual arthritis treatments of exercise, physical therapy, and painkillers don't work as well for people with scoliosis as for those without.

When thoracic curves progress beyond 50 degrees, shifting ribs can constrict the heart or lungs. This causes shortness of breath, low energy, or a general sense of being unwell. These effects aren't usually severe until curves reach 70 to 100 degrees. A small number of adults with curves greater than 100 degrees die from restrictive lung disease. Children with IIS or JIS whose curves reach 50 degrees before age five can also die if compression prevents their lungs from developing properly.

Progression slows dramatically when growth is complete, but two thirds of curves continue worsening after patients reach adulthood. Cobb angles above 50 degrees are at highest risk of this, and there's some evidence curve pattern and poor physical fitness may also be factors, especially for women. Save all your teen X-rays so further changes to your curve can be easily measured in adulthood.

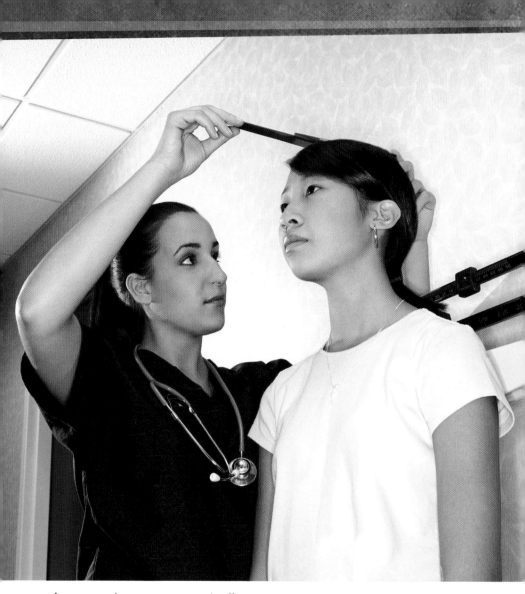

A progressive curve can actually make you shorter over time.

ESTIMATING YOUR RISK

Natural history is the progression your AIS will follow if you never receive treatment. A person's natural history can't usually be predicted with certainty, but a number of risk factors for progression have been identified. Age at diagnosis is most important because rapid progression occurs during growth spurts. In adolescents, curves may worsen by as much as 20 to 30 degrees each year.[3] Therefore, the younger you are when diagnosed, the higher your risk of progression.

Curve severity and curve pattern play a role in progression, too. The higher the Cobb angle at diagnosis, the higher the risk of progression. Only 10 to 15 percent of adolescents with Cobb angles below 25 progress.[4] Thoracic curves are more likely to progress than any other type and are most likely to result in dangerous complications.

Gender is also a risk factor. Girls have a five to ten times higher risk of curve progression than boys.[5] Teens with starting curves above 30 degrees, however, are equally likely to

THE ECONOMICS OF SCOLIOSIS

Because it's hard to identify low-risk patients accurately, doctors monitor as if everyone is at high risk for progression. Therefore, many kids with AIS endure unnecessary monitoring and treatment, creating needless anxiety for them and their families.

In the United States, AIS has a total impact of 600,000 doctor's visits, 30,000 brace applications, and 18,000 spinal fusion surgeries annually.[6] The total economic cost of the disorder may be as high as $4 billion a year.[7]

worsen regardless of gender.[8] The more risk factors you have, the greater your total risk. For example, girls ages 10 to 12 with curves more than 30 degrees at diagnosis have an overall progression risk of 90 to 100 percent.[9]

CHOOSING NOT TO TREAT

Family doctors may not be aware of the risks of curve progression, so always get a specialist's opinion before deciding whether or how to treat your AIS. Consulting multiple specialists is even better. For small, low-risk curves, the standard treatment is observation. This regular monitoring allows doctors to catch progression in the early stages so it can be treated before leading to health complications.

SCOLIOSIS AND BREAST CANCER

Girls diagnosed with AIS between 1920 and 1989 are 1.7 times more likely to die of breast cancer than women without scoliosis. The reason? Repeated X-rays used during observation and treatment. In this time period, the average teen with scoliosis had 24.7 X-rays, and 15 percent of patients were scanned 50 or more times. Cancer risk increased with increasing radiation exposure and was highest for women diagnosed in the 1940s to 1950s.[10]

Modern X-ray technology uses much less radiation than in the past. Still, doctors often order posterior views to increase the distance between a girl's breasts and the beam, and protective lead shields are always used. The increase in cancer risk with AIS is just two cases per 1 million women.[11]

Because scoliosis treatments have their own drawbacks, many patients decide not to treat even after progression is observed. This is a valid choice, but it also has consequences. If you change your mind later on, bracing or surgery might be less successful. Whichever path you choose, be certain you're motivated by information rather than emotion.

ASK YOURSELF THIS

- *Do you have a support group or close friends you can speak to about your scoliosis concerns?*

- *Based on the known risk factors, is your chance of curve progression low or high?*

- *What worries you more—health complications or the fact your asymmetry might become more noticeable?*

- *Have you avoided treatment for your scoliosis? If so, why?*

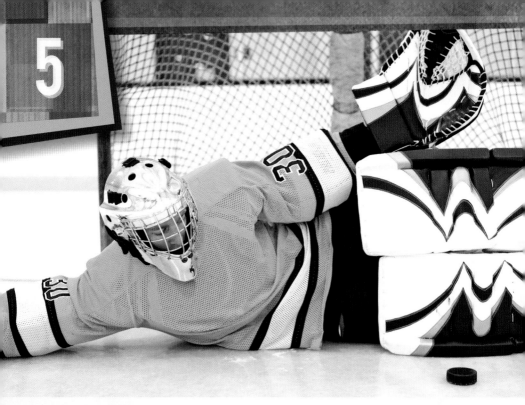

BRACING FOR THE WORST

X ander stared straight ahead. The orthotist was scanning his spine, and he was ready to bolt out of the door as soon as she was finished.

Grams watched, her gray hair tightly knotted and a steely glint in her eyes. He had tried

It's possible to find a balance between bracing and still being involved in your favorite activities.

to tell her he didn't want to wear a brace—it wasn't likely it would fit under his hockey pads anyway—but she wouldn't listen. She treated his crooked spine as a personal affront, and she was bound and determined to get him back on the straight and narrow. Literally.

"All right, that's it!" the orthotist said. "That didn't take very long, did it? This 3-D scan will help us fit you for a brace that will be tailored perfectly for your spine. And we'll have all of this in a permanent electronic file, so it will be easy to track any changes. Now I know a brace isn't exactly what you had in mind, but it's important to wear it as often as prescribed if you want to see any results."

Grams kept surprisingly quiet until the ride home. Naturally, she started in as soon as we closed our car doors. "You remember what the doctor said?"

"Yes, Grams."

"It won't work if you don't wear it."

"I know, Grams."

"I think you should give up hockey until the treatment's done."

"Grams!" Xander snapped. "You know I want to play for the NHL—you think I'll have a shot if I take two years off?"

BRACING: A HISTORY

Modern braces are major improvements compared to historical treatments, which included:

- Breathing exercises, such as singing loudly
- Bed rest for two to three years
- Metal corsets weighing 20 to 30 pounds (9 to 14 kg)
- Plaster body casts that couldn't be removed
- Braces that caused pain if the patient didn't actively stand up straight
- Stretching using weights, pulleys, and ropes

"You think you'll have a shot if you're bent in half?"

Xander glared at his feet. He didn't care how many doctors Gram dragged him to. He felt fine, so it couldn't be as bad as they wanted him to think. "I'm not risking my dream for this," he said.

"Then you'll wear that thing every single second you're not at the rink."

Xander snorted. They'd just see about that, wouldn't they?

TO BRACE OR NOT TO BRACE

Scoliosis curves progress because unbalanced pressure on the vertebrae causes uneven growth. Custom-built scoliosis braces reverse these pressures, slowing growth on the outside of your curve and speeding it up on the inside. This allows your spine to stabilize naturally.

The treatment's goal is to prevent progression, and in doing so, avoid the need for surgery. Braces are not cures. In most cases, they will not correct curves you already have. With this in mind, bracing is a good option for you if:

- Your curve is between 20 and 40 degrees and you're at risk of progression.

- You have at least 18 months of growing left, providing opportunity for the treatment to work.

- Your apex is below T4. Bracing is less successful for curves involving neck vertebrae.

- You're committed to wearing the brace for 21 to 23 hours every day until you finish growing, removing it only for showers and sports.

- You're happy with the way you look, despite any existing asymmetry.

IS BRACING RIGHT FOR YOU?

Bracing is the only nonsurgical treatment shown to stop curve progression. However, it probably won't work if your home environment is not supportive, you're unwilling to comply with your bracing schedule, or you're overweight, preventing the brace from delivering adequate force through your body's soft tissue.

Another consideration is young children sometimes develop chest and rib deformations from the pressure braces exert on soft, developing bones. This isn't usually a problem for teens, but you should discuss any concerns with your doctor before starting treatment.

A BRACE FOR EVERY BODY

Scoliosis braces use custom-designed pads to push the lateral curves of your spine toward the center of your body. The pads may also provide turning force, counteracting any vertebral rotation. Brace design depends on your curve and lifestyle. The most common models include the Milwaukee, the Boston, the Charleston, and the SpineCor.

Designed in 1954, the Milwaukee is the first modern scoliosis brace and has the highest success rate when worn as directed. Rigid bars connect a plastic hip girdle to a metal neck ring, stretching the body upward, while straps and pads redirect the spine. Because the Milwaukee is the least comfortable and hardest brace to hide, many teens refuse to wear it. These days,

BRAIST: THE BRACING FOR ADOLESCENT IDIOPATHIC SCOLIOSIS TRIAL

To gather definitive data on bracing for scoliosis, doctors at 25 hospitals in the United States and Canada conducted the world's first controlled clinical trial. The study compared full-time use of Boston braces to similar patients who chose not to be treated. The braces included temperature sensors that accurately measured hours of wear, and teens in both groups also supplied data on how AIS affected their physical functioning, self-esteem, and quality of life. The trial ended early in January 2013 after bracing was proven significantly effective in reducing study participants' curve progressions.

it's used only for high, thoracic curves that can't be treated with other braces.

The Boston is a plastic shell with corrective pads inside. The brace begins at the pelvis and ends below the arms. It's less bulky than the Milwaukee, making it easier to disguise under clothing.

The Charleston is used for flexible C-curves only. It stretches the body toward the outside of the curve. This forced bend means the Charleston can only be worn while sleeping.

Lastly, the SpineCor brace has a plastic pelvic piece similar to the others, but it applies corrective pressure using strong rubber bands. Unfortunately, SpineCor seems to work only for young patients with small, flexible curves. For curves exceeding 20 degrees, a rigid brace is a better choice.

DOES BRACING ACTUALLY WORK?

Large-scale research studies comparing the results of bracing versus observation have never been done. This is partly because bracing has been the standard treatment for 2,000 years and partly because it's not ethical for scientists to deny treatment to patients in a study when there's already some evidence it helps.

In the absence of properly controlled research, however, some doctors question whether bracing for scoliosis is truly an

EXERCISING WHILE BRACED

In addition to its general health benefits, exercise during bracing helps prevent your back muscles from shrinking. A physical therapist can teach you movements that will support your treatment. Most of the physical activities you already enjoy can also be done while wearing a brace, but you should remove it for swimming and contact sports, in which a collision with your hardware could injure someone else. See your doctor with questions about specific activities.

improvement compared to doing nothing at all. It doesn't help that the data we do have contradicts itself. Some studies show teens who wear braces are just as likely to wind up having surgery as teens who don't, while others conclude braced patients are less likely to need surgery than those who refuse treatment.

The latest evidence suggests the degree to which patients follow the recommended wear schedule explains these contradictions. A study using sensors inside the braces proved even though most teens claimed they were following instructions, only 15 percent of them were fully compliant. Of this 15 percent, only 11 percent had curves that progressed during treatment.[1] However, progression occurred in 56 percent of patients who wore their braces less than recommended.[2] Other human studies

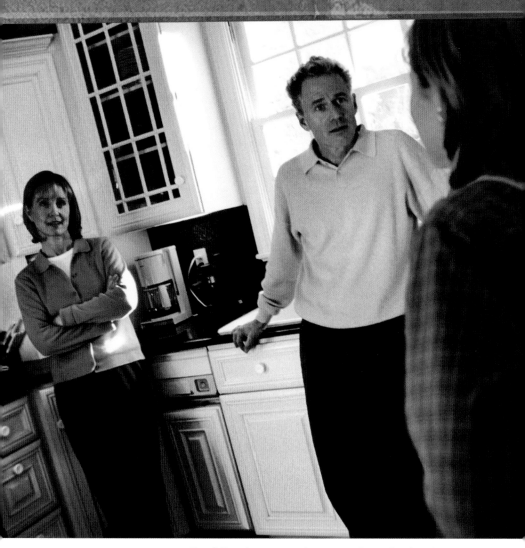

*Deciding to wear a brace and continuing to wear
it are common battles for teens with scoliosis.*

also suggest dosage is everything, and recent
animal research confirms part-time bracing (for
example, nighttime braces) is of very little value.

The goal of a brace is halting progression,
but only you can decide whether not getting
worse is enough motivation for you to wear your
brace as directed. Unfortunately, many teens

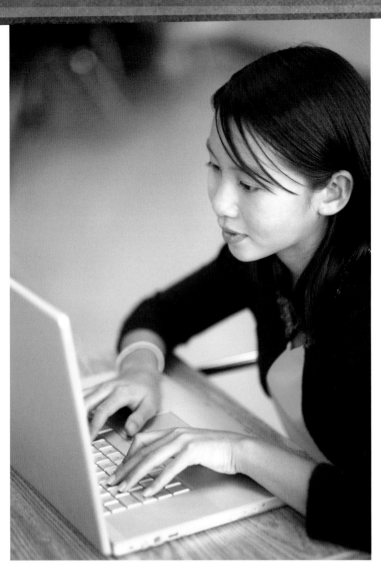

Do your own research to see how bracing has or hasn't worked for others.

whose braces worked still go on to have surgery. If you're already unhappy with your appearance, you're most likely to fall into this group. If you don't think you'll be satisfied even if the brace treatment is successful, talk to your doctor about surgery instead.

ASK YOURSELF THIS

- *If your doctor recommended years of bracing, how would you react?*

- *Does it surprise you some doctors are debating the usefulness of bracing? How does this affect your attitude toward the treatment?*

- *Do you think Xander's bracing is likely to be successful?*

- *What is your goal for treatment? Have you considered whether bracing would actually meet that goal?*

- *Could you stick to a daily exercise plan if your doctor recommended it?*

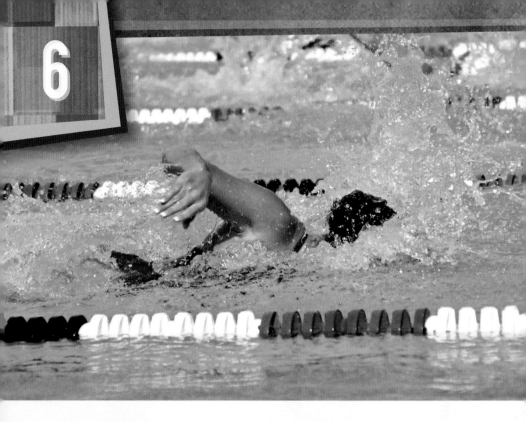

COPING WITH BRACE WEAR

Maddy shimmied out of her swimsuit and took a closer look at the rub mark on her hip. She didn't realize her brace had chafed until she hit the pool and it had started to sting. The raw spot wasn't too bad, but she'd ask Dad to call the orthotist anyway.

She'd grown so much over the last couple of months, it was probably time for an adjustment.

"Mad, what's the hold up?" Liv yelled from down the row. "You want me to strap you in or what?"

"Be right there!" Maddy buttoned her jeans and pulled on her undershirt before leaving the stall, then positioned her brace and turned away so Liv could fasten it behind her. Maddy had heard some braces closed in the front, but her doctor insisted on the Boston model. At first, she was worried about inconveniencing people, but her fellow teammates seemed to get a kick out of helping her dress after practice. It didn't hurt that she was still the fastest swimmer on the team.

"You'll never guess what Jake told me," Liv said as they headed for the street. "Tony's going to ask you out!"

"I can't go out with anyone," Maddy protested.

"Why not?"

Maddy made a vague "I'm such a freak" gesture, and Liv burst out laughing. "Come on, Mad, if the abs of plastic don't bother Tony, why should they bother you?"

Liv was right, of course. It was just that Maddy had pretty much figured no one would be interested in the girl in the iron maiden. Now that someone might be, she wasn't sure if she should be excited or just nervous. "But what would I wear?" she asked weakly.

Liv laughed again, hooking her arm through Maddy's. "Leave that part to me."

THE FIRST FEW WEEKS

If you've committed to a brace, you may have second thoughts the minute you first put it on. The brace will squeeze and poke you and make you feel as if you're in a cage. You might have trouble bending down, taking deep breaths, or getting comfortable enough to sleep. If your curve is high enough to need a Milwaukee, the neck ring will also make it difficult to turn or bend your head.

Try thinking of your brace as a pair of shoes needing breaking in. For the first week or so, wear it until you can't stand it, then take it off. Rest for up to one hour, then put it back on. Some teens report that after adapting to

HANDLING QUESTIONS

It may not be possible to hide your brace from classmates and teachers, and avoiding the issue can lead to unpleasant rumors or speculation. Try being open about your condition and be willing to answer people's questions. This increases social acceptance, helping you feel less alone. You may even find people admire your courage and determination.

the brace, they're actually more comfortable with it than without.

Besides breaking it in, your brace should not be painful. Try it on before leaving the orthotist's and speak up about sharp edges or discomfort. If new issues develop after the initial fitting, you may have grown enough to need a bigger size. At three- or four-month checkups, the orthotist will address any problems and may also tighten the brace to increase the force it applies to your curve. Expect that you'll need a few days to get used to any adjustments.

"I wore turtlenecks all year long, even in hot, muggy weather, in the hope that nobody would find out my secret. But guess what? Most of my friends and acquaintances knew I was wearing a brace, and frankly, they didn't care if they saw a little metal encircling my neck. And after sweating it out for several months, I finally decided that my undercover act just wasn't worth the bother. I wore anything I felt like wearing, including V-neck T-shirts and bare-midriff tops! This 'flaunting' of my brace made me feel better about myself—I was proud that I could endure wearing this contraption. I was showing the world that I could handle it. And that's something that not everyone can do!"

—*A teen girl with AIS*[1]

SURVIVING THE TREATMENT

Patients have developed a series of strategies for coping with brace wear. Make life easier with these time-tested tips: It's normal for muscles to ache as your body adjusts to a straighter position, but consult your doctor if you're too uncomfortable. Protect your skin by wearing a tight, seamless top beneath the brace; girls should choose sports bras without hooks or underwires. Natural fibers such as cotton are best. Never use body lotion on skin covered by the brace. The softer your skin, the worse the chafing. Treat sore spots with rubbing alcohol or Toughskin. Long hair and Milwaukee braces don't mix. Avoid getting tangled in the neck ring by pinning up your locks. While braced, you may have to squat to pick objects up or try out a new

DRESS TO IMPRESS

Wearing a brace doesn't have to make you a fashion victim. AIS patients recommend:

- Elastic waist pants or skirts one size too big to fit over the pelvic girdle
- Low waists and hipster jeans to lengthen the look of your torso
- Underpants that fit over the brace to make bathroom breaks simpler
- Dark colors, small patterns or textures, and layers to disguise asymmetry or lumps
- A good tailor who can add hidden pads to suits or formal dresses to balance out your shape
- Accessories, such as drop belts, scarves, and jewelry, that draw attention away from areas you want to hide
- Heels below 1 to 2 inches (3 to 5 cm), minimizing unnecessary pressure on your spine
- Clothes that make you feel comfortable and confident, regardless of whether they hide your brace

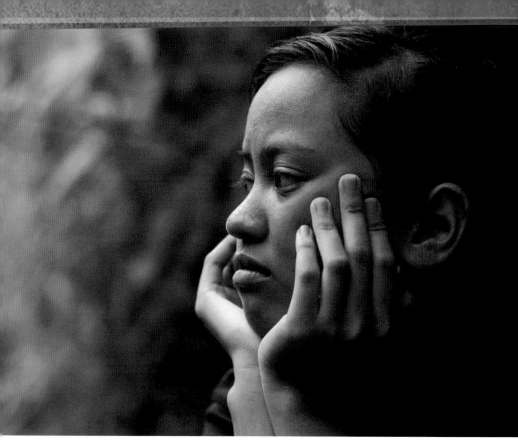

There is a strong possibility feelings of anxiety and isolation will develop at the beginning of treatment.

sleeping position. If sleeping's uncomfortable, use body pillows for added support. Clean your brace with a damp, soapy cloth, and if you're creative, feel free to decorate it!

HAVING A LIFE

Body image and peer acceptance have a bigger impact on people's mental health during the teen years than at any other stage of life. Scoliosis and its treatments can make patients feel embarrassed, awkward, and even unattractive, impacting their social relationships and self-esteem.

In one survey, 84 percent of families said the first six months were the worst, while their teen adjusted to the physical and emotional challenges of brace wear.[2] It does get easier, however, and in the long-term, most teens braced for AIS have the same self-esteem and quality of life as teens without scoliosis. Braced patients also tend to have higher self-esteem and life satisfaction than AIS patients who refuse treatment.

When your bones are almost finished growing—usually at Risser 4—you'll begin weaning off the brace. This involves gradually reducing your daily wear time until you're ready to stop bracing entirely. After each reduction, your doctor will check to ensure your spine is maintaining its position. If so, you'll continue

DATING AND SEXUALITY

Thirty percent of adults who wore braces for AIS said they eliminated all social activities during treatment, and 40 percent believed bracing had limited their opportunities for romantic relationships.[3] It's natural to worry about your crush's perceptions of your scoliosis or your brace, but if you catch yourself thinking "Nobody will ever be attracted to me," stop right there! Besides being untrue, these negative beliefs undermine the very confidence and self-esteem that make you attractive. Discuss concerns about sexuality with fellow patients, your doctor, or another trusted adult. And remember: the only limitations scoliosis imposes are the ones you place on yourself.

cutting back. If your curve progresses, however, your wear schedule will increase or your doctor will recommend surgery.

If you're having trouble adjusting to treatment, the best coping strategy is talking about it—with family, friends, or other scoliosis patients who know exactly what you're going through. One study showed teens who knew someone else undergoing bracing were much less unhappy about wearing braces.

CONFIDE IN OTHERS

AIS patients agree talking is key to successfully coping with and treating scoliosis. When you're ready:

- Join a local chapter of the National Scoliosis Association. Many areas have meetings just for teens. If a group is not already available, find out how to start your own.
- Look for online chat rooms and support groups.
- Ask your doctor for the contact information of previous patients.
- Lean on family, friends, or religious groups for support.
- For really difficult emotions, a psychologist, counselor, or social worker can help.

Your treatment's impact on your life depends largely upon your personality and situation. Problem-solvers with supportive family and friends find bracing has little impact on their mental and emotional health. In contrast, bracing may seriously threaten the happiness and self-esteem of teens who are hard on

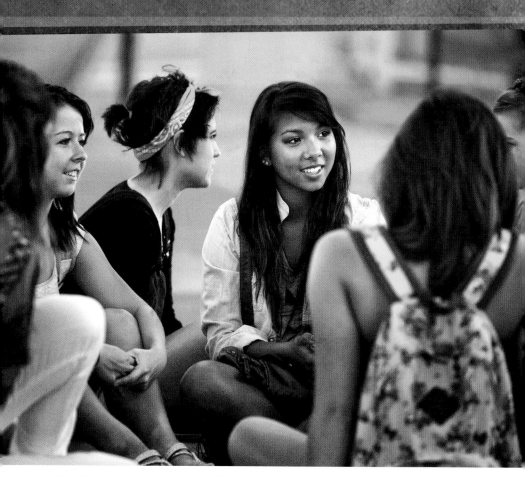

Confide in friends you trust if you are having issues adjusting to your treatment.

themselves, obsess over setbacks, or place a lot of importance on other people's opinions.

Successful bracing requires commitment—both daily and for the months and years of growing still ahead of you. It's difficult to accept immediate feelings of limitation in exchange for a long-term payoff that's not guaranteed. If you can complete this treatment, be proud of your accomplishment. If you're among the many teens who can't, don't judge yourself harshly.

You are not a failure, and you are not destroying your own health. You may, however, be facing scoliosis surgery.

ASK YOURSELF THIS

- *What could you do to support a friend who's being treated for scoliosis?*

- *What physical aspect of brace treatment would be most difficult for you?*

- *Are you a problem-solver, or do you tend to dwell? How do you think your approach to life in general would affect your response to bracing?*

- *How would you handle questions about your brace? What could you do to help your teachers or peers understand and accept your condition?*

- *How would you feel if bracing did not stop the progression of your curve?*

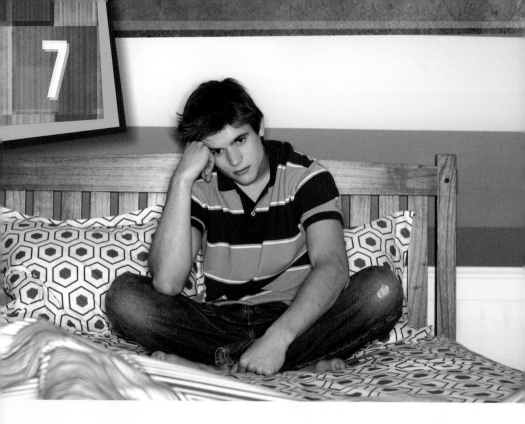

SURGERIES FOR SCOLIOSIS

Colton sat cross-legged on the middle of his bed, the pile of brochures and printouts fanned out in front of him. He had not been able to get over his body's betrayal.

Colton had worn his brace religiously for three years. He had a lumbar curve, and his doctor had told him his chance of progression was low—that the brace was mostly a precaution. But Colton hadn't taken any risks. He wanted to be a professional dancer, and a mobile spine was definitely a requirement. He wore the brace every second he wasn't at rehearsal, and quite a few times during, because he believed he could avoid the surgery that would decimate his dreams.

It turned out his curve had other plans.

All the surgeons his parents consulted said the same thing. He'd still be able to dance after the fusion—just not professionally. They were also united in the opinion that his 50-degree curve would keep getting worse until they operated. But every one of them proposed a slightly different surgical approach, and Colton didn't know how he'd be able to choose between them when no matter what he did, the end result would be the same.

His big sister knocked on the door and poked her head in. "Still deciding?"

Colton shrugged, avoiding her eyes. "Does it really make a difference?"

"Oh, come on, Colton." She crossed the room and perched next to him on the bed, sympathy in her eyes. "I know it doesn't feel like it right now, but there is more to life than dance."

Colton wasn't so sure.

SPINAL FUSION SURGERY

There is a 10 to 25 percent chance your curve will progress despite bracing.[1] If you've reached 50 degrees as Colton had, you're at high risk of continued progression during adulthood, too. Most specialists will recommend spinal fusion surgery to avoid health complications associated with severe curves. Vertebrae that are surgically fused can no longer grow or twist, preventing progression. Surgery is also the only treatment for AIS that straightens existing curves, reducing any asymmetry you might already have.

USING SHAPE-MEMORY METAL

Two of the downsides of spinal fusion surgery are loss of flexibility and the extreme forces required to instantly correct curves. An alternative being tested is gradual correction, which uses nitinol, or shape-memory metal. Nitinol can be bent when it's cool but regains its original shape when heated to body temperature. In 2012, researchers implanted nitinol wires on the spines of scoliotic rats. As the wires gradually straightened, they applied gentle force to correct the rats' curves without affecting mobility. On average, curves improved from 79.3 degrees to 8.7 degrees.[2]

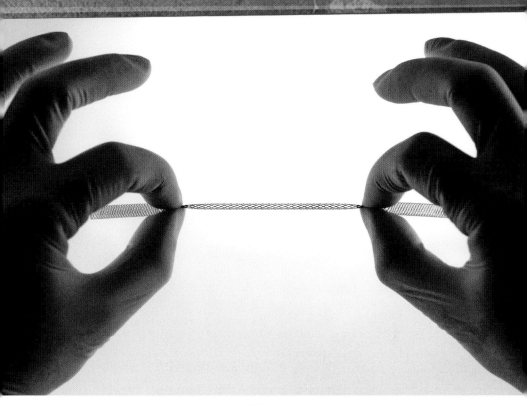

Nitinol, a shape-memory metal made of nickel and titanium, has proven successful in dramatically reducing spinal curves in rats.

BASICS OF FUSION SURGERY

Dr. Russell Hibbs performed the first spinal fusion in 1911. The procedure took a full year because Dr. Hibbs could fuse just two or three vertebrae in a single surgery. After each session, patients spent six to eight weeks in the hospital wearing a body cast. Today, fusion surgery takes just four to 12 hours, and patients are back home within a week.

Spinal fusion involves several steps. First, the surgeon makes one or more incisions to expose the spine. The outer layer of

GROWING RODS FOR GROWING KIDS

JIS can cause serious health problems long before growth is complete. In these cases, surgeons delay fusion using growing rods. Implanted on the spine, the rods hold the vertebrae straight, creating space for immature lungs to finish developing. Every six months, the surgeon makes a new incision to access the rods and lengthens them for the next stage of growth. After skeletal maturity, the rods are removed and fusion surgery is completed.

the vertebrae is removed, revealing the living, growing bone beneath. Next, bone grafts are cut into small strips and packed over the vertebrae to be fused. This is similar to joining two foam blocks by wrapping them with papier-mâché. Lastly, to hold the fused vertebrae in place while healing, the surgeon installs metal instrumentation.

Instrumentation can include rods that winch the ends of the spine apart, as a car jack, or a system of wires, hooks, and screws which rotate and secure the vertebrae in their new alignment. This hardware is usually left in place even after healing is complete.

For patients with rib humps, doctors may also recommend thoracoplasty. This surgery involves removing a few inches of length from the center of the affected ribs, causing them to settle down into the chest. The cut ends heal together within six to 12 weeks, and the

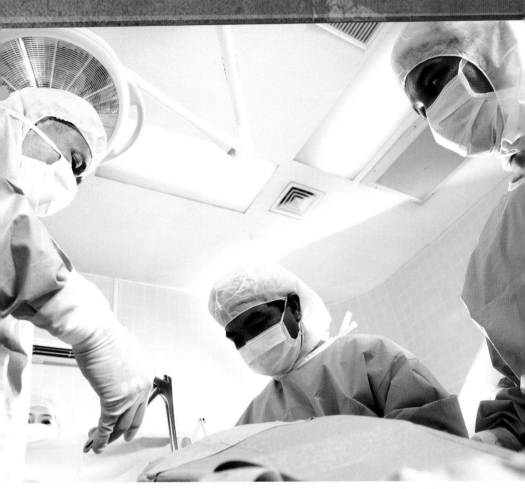

*Take the time to research and talk to
your family and physician before deciding
if fusion surgery is right for you.*

rib hump is usually smaller by approximately
70 percent.[3]

WHAT YOU NEED TO KNOW

Depending on ability and experience, different
doctors may recommend different surgical
approaches for the same patient. Always get
at least two opinions before making a decision.

CHOOSING A SURGEON

Your surgeon's skill is critical to the success of your operation, and you need to trust whomever you choose. Ask your surgeon about his or her specialized training and qualifications for scoliosis surgery, how many scoliosis surgeries he or she performs each year, and if you can talk to former patients who had similar curves. If you live in a small town, you might need to travel to find a qualified surgeon. Start your search by visiting the Scoliosis Research Society at www.srs.org.

Consider all aspects of the proposed surgery, such as the source of your bone graft. If your doctor harvests your hip or rib bones for the graft, pain at the harvest site may be worse than the pain in your spine. On the other hand, your body may reject bone grafts taken from an organ donor. Point of entry is important, too. Surgeons can reach your spine from the back or the side. Side-access involves deflating one of your lungs, and therefore has a higher risk of complications. For large, inflexible curves, however, both routes might be needed, so always ask surgeons to explain their choice. Find out what kinds of hardware your surgeon will use and why. Ask about material as well. If you're allergic to the nickel found in stainless steel, you'll need titanium implants instead.

Measurement errors in Cobb angle can influence surgical recommendations, so make

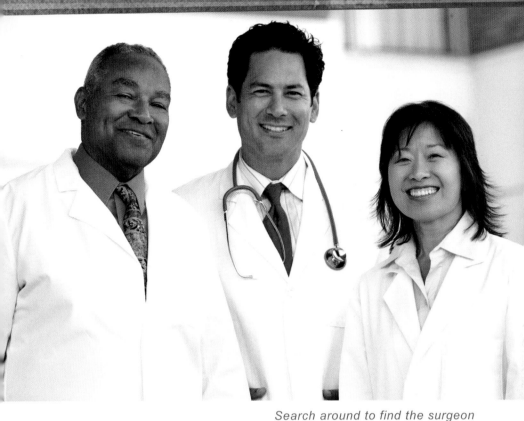

Search around to find the surgeon who best suits your needs.

sure the numbers are consistent. Consider what life will be like afterward, as well. If you enjoy activities requiring a wide range of motion, flexibility after surgery will be an important consideration. Most of your movement comes from your lumbar vertebrae, which cannot bend if fused.

For many teens, the cosmetic effects of scoliosis are more important than health complications. It's important to recognize surgery cannot give you a completely straight spine. In fact, large corrections can only be achieved by applying extreme force, which can crack vertebrae or cause spinal cord injury. Overcorrecting can also cause vertebrae that weren't fused to compensate by developing brand-new curves. In most cases, surgeons can safely correct curves by up to 70 to 80 percent.[4] Discuss cosmetic concerns with your surgeon before the procedure—you'll be happier with the outcome if you start with realistic expectations.

COMPLICATIONS AND OUTCOMES

All surgeries have risks, and spinal fusion is no exception. You'll need to weigh these risks against any benefits the procedure may offer. Complications specific to scoliosis surgery include:

- *Crankshafting.* If you need surgery before you finish growing, your surgeon will fuse both sides of your vertebrae. This prevents crankshafting—continued growth on the unfused side, which deforms vertebrae and creates new curves.

- *Infection.* To lessen your risk of infection after surgery, your doctor will prescribe antibiotics before, during, and after the procedure.

- *Pain caused by hardware.* This is rare, but may require a second surgery to remove instrumentation.

- *Progression above or below your fusion.* If your doctor does a short fusion to avoid lost flexibility, unfused vertebrae might still shift over time.

- *Blood loss and breathing problems.* This is more common with rib surgery and in patients with asthma.

- *Nerve damage or paralysis.* Doctors monitor your nerve function during surgery, and with an experienced surgeon, this risk is almost zero.

STAPLES AND TETHERS

Doctors are using the principles of bracing—manipulating rates of bone growth—to develop new surgical treatments for scoliosis. In one procedure, vertebrae are stapled along the outer edge of the curve, slowing growth on that side. For kids with curves under 20 degrees and at least one year of growth remaining, the success rate is 86 percent.[5] However, since kids with small curves usually have low risk of progression anyway, it's not yet clear how effective this technique really is.

A second technique, called tethering, involves anchoring a stretchy plastic cord to the ends of the curve along the convex side. More research is still needed; as of 2012, only 20 patients had received this surgery.[6]

The goal of both techniques is to correct curves early, before the more invasive spinal fusions become necessary. Since these techniques don't restrict flexibility, they're promising for active teens who want to maintain full range of motion.

OBESITY INCREASES RISK

Teens who are obese have both a higher risk of developing AIS and less chance of successful bracing.[8] If you're in this situation, surgery may be your only option. Fusion works just as well for obese teens, and complications are just as rare as for kids with healthy weights. However, the surgery often takes longer, causing patients to lose more blood. It's also harder to deliver painkillers directly to the spines of obese patients. Unfortunately, taking heavy-duty painkillers by mouth instead increases the risk of breathing problems after surgery and may lengthen hospital stays. Discuss any concerns with your doctor before scheduling surgery.

Statistically, teens have many fewer complications than adults, especially if they're in good physical shape and eat a healthy diet.[7] In addition, curves become less flexible with age, limiting the amount of correction a surgeon can achieve. If you're considering surgery, these are good reasons not to delay.

However, keep in mind spinal fusion is only medically necessary if you're experiencing heart and lung problems, severe pain, or can't complete basic life tasks. Unless your curve is progressing rapidly, you have time to consider your options, goals, and risks before committing to a procedure. Wait until you're completely convinced surgery is the best choice for you.

ASK YOURSELF THIS

- *What is your main reason for considering scoliosis surgery?*

- *Could you accept the loss of flexibility resulting from spinal fusion?*

- *How would you feel about accepting a bone graft from another person, living or dead?*

- *Does the idea of permanent metal implants disturb you?*

- *What improvement in your health or appearance would be necessary to make the risks of surgery worthwhile?*

- *Would you feel better about receiving the well-tested spinal fusion or one of the new methods doctors are currently developing?*

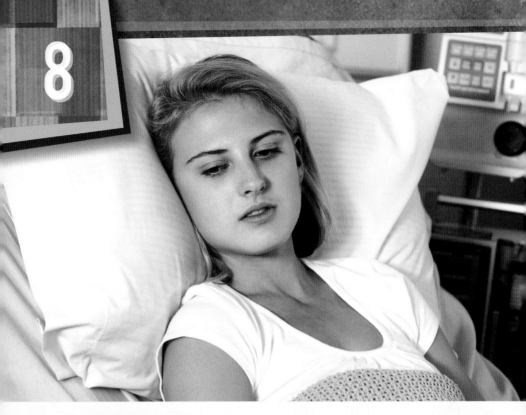

STANDING TALLER: BEFORE AND AFTER SURGERY

"**H**ow are we feeling today?"

Bree cracked an eyelid, resisting the urge to point out that was a silly question. It was her third day after surgery, and the only word for the way she felt was "gross." It had been way too long since her last shower, and her hip ached where the surgeon had harvested the bone grafts. She kept using the pain pump, even though the meds made her groggy. Bree had a vague notion that when her boyfriend David came to visit, she had asked him to catch her a purple monkey. She really hoped that part was just a dream.

The nurse was waiting for a reply, and Bree tilted her head. "Okay, I guess," she whispered—her throat was still sore.

"That's good," the nurse replied, "because it's time to walk."

Bree wasn't sure about this plan, but she was too weak to fend off the nurse and the entirely too cheerful physical therapist who joined them. They helped her swing her legs over the edge of the bed and paused until her vision stopped swimming. Then they got her on her feet and held her steady while she tried to remember how to stand.

Supported on either side, Bree took a few steps. Her brain knew she was straighter now, but her body was convinced she was leaning to the left. And something else was off. Why were her feet so far away?

"Oh my gosh," Bree said. She couldn't tell if she was shaking with exhaustion or excitement. "Did I get *taller*?"

The women laughed as they helped her back to bed. Bree grinned. She couldn't wait for David to get back—for the first time ever, she wouldn't have to look up to meet his eyes.

PREPARING FOR SURGERY

Because scoliosis surgery is only rarely an emergency, you can choose the best time of year to have it. Recovery takes several weeks, so pick a date that won't interfere with school or other important life events. Before you're officially approved, you'll have to complete a series of medical tests. These include fresh X-rays used in planning the fusion and a physical to check your general health. You might also be asked to donate blood, which

PAYING FOR SURGERY

In the United States, surgery for AIS may cost anywhere from $75,000 to $300,000.[1] In one survey, 53 percent of families said additional income was needed to cover these expenses, although only 26 percent considered it a problem.[2]

As part of your preparation, ask about surgery costs and payment options. If you don't have health insurance, a surgeon who works at a teaching or research hospital may be able to arrange partial coverage. If you're under the age of 18, the Shriners Hospital group might also be willing to pay for your treatment.

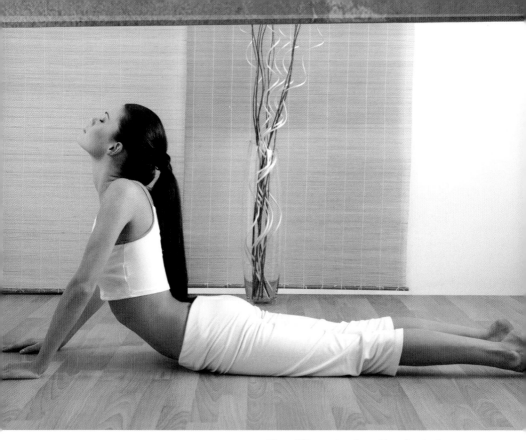

Try different relaxation techniques, such as meditation or yoga, to help calm you down before surgery.

will be given back to you if you need it during surgery.

The rest of the preparation is in your hands. Good health speeds recovery, so stay active and eat well. If you have acne on your back, treat it to reduce the risk of an infected incision. Stop taking painkillers two weeks in advance, as they can inhibit bone fusion or cause excess bleeding during surgery. And lastly, pack a bag with slippers, a robe, toiletries, and any other items you'll need during your hospital stay.

As much as you may want surgery, preparing for it can be very stressful. Ask other surgery patients what to expect. See if you can skip school, work, or chores the day before—do something fun to put you in a positive mindset for the challenge ahead.

AT THE HOSPITAL

If you're nervous the morning of the procedure, ask whether your family can join you until you're sedated. You won't feel anything during surgery, and when you wake up, you won't be allowed visitors for the first few hours. This is actually a good thing—between the anesthesia and the pain medication, you might behave strangely or say things you normally wouldn't. To avoid potential awkwardness, it's okay to ask visitors to wait a few days until the drugs have cleared your system.

SURGERY Q & A

Many frequently asked surgery questions relate to implanted hardware. In case you've wondered:

- You probably won't feel it, unless pressure is applied directly over the metal.
- Instrumentation needs to be removed only if it causes problems.
- It weighs 1 to 3 pounds (0.5 to 1.5 kg).
- It won't rust.
- It will not set off most airport metal detectors. When traveling, pack a letter from your doctor and be prepared to show your scar just in case.

Grogginess, disorientation, nausea, and stiffness are all normal following surgery. So is pain, which you'll feel in your back, throat, or areas where bone grafts were harvested. You should also expect some general achiness as your muscles adapt to your spine's new position. If your doctor gives you a personally controlled analgesic (PCA) for regulating your own painkillers, don't hesitate to use it. These pain pumps are computer controlled, so it's impossible to overdose.

You'll be expected to get out of bed within two or three days after surgery. Walking will feel strange at first. Your legs may be weak, and you might be convinced you're leaning when you're actually standing straighter than before. A straightened spine will also make you up to four inches (10 cm) taller, so don't be surprised if it takes time to adjust to your new center of gravity.

RETURNING HOME: PHYSICAL HEALING

If everything goes smoothly, you'll be home within five to seven days. Make recovery easier by moving important items to your level of reach to eliminate bending and stretching and wear button-up shirts until you're comfortable raising your arms.

The more you move, the faster you'll heal, so try to increase the distance you walk a little every day. Rest when you need to, and don't be discouraged if you suddenly feel worse after several days of improvement. This is normal and passes quickly. You should call your doctor immediately, however, if you have: signs of infection—a fever or incision that splits, oozes, or smells bad; severe, persistent pain and meds aren't helping; or numbness, tingling, or weakness that might suggest nerve damage.

BACK TO NORMAL

Recovering from surgery can be very emotional. It's natural to become anxious or depressed, or to feel frightened when people touch your healing back. Call your doctor with questions, and draw on friends, family, or other sources of support if you're overwhelmed by difficult emotions.

On the other hand, some patients find physical appearance improvement boosts their happiness and self-confidence. If you fall into this group, you'll be tempted to launch back in

"Luckily for me, I think in retrospect, I probably had the best situation because they found [my AIS] at a point where nothing could be done *except* the operation. I really would have hated it if they'd found it at maybe 30 degrees and I would have had to wear a brace for five or six years. I think that would have been the worst. For the kids I know who've had the operation *after* bracing, it was this incredibly liberating experience."

—*Susannah, an AIS patient*[3]

to life as quickly as possible. Remember to pace yourself. Your friends can visit as soon as you get home, but don't plan to go out until you're off painkillers and feeling relatively normal.

You'll be cleared for school within two to four weeks, but it might be longer before you can carry a backpack comfortably—keeping a set of books at school and at home will help. Avoid contact sports and high-impact activities such as running or jumping for four to six months while your bone grafts finish fusing. And even if you've never felt better, save the skydiving for your one year anniversary!

ASK YOURSELF THIS

- *What type of treatment better suits your personality—bracing or surgery?*

- *What scares you most about fusion surgery? How could you deal with that fear?*

- *What preparations would you need to make to feel confident and in control during recovery?*

- *What limits or liberties would a successful fusion surgery place on your life?*

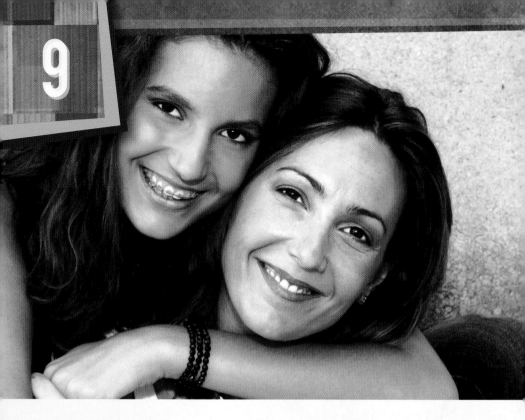

TWISTS IN THE ROAD: LIFESTYLE AND LIFE

Harper grabbed her mat and darted out to the car. Mom had the engine running, and she pulled away before Harper had even fastened her seat belt. She didn't mind, though—she didn't want to be late, either.

They had started going to yoga classes together as soon as Harper's doctor told her she could finally stop wearing the brace. Harper loved yoga because it made her feel tall and powerful. Mom loved it because the poses helped with her stiffness and pain. The part they both loved best, though, was that they were sharing something. Before Harper found out she had inherited her mother's scoliosis, the two of them barely talked at all.

After class, their muscles all warm and wobbly, they went for ice cream. Harper talked about the experiment she was working on for the science fair and her hopes about it taking her to Nationals. Not to mention Yale. Blushing like a teenager, Mom reported her plans for her first date with Andrew. It was so amazing to Harper their lives weren't about her scoliosis anymore. She was happy her mom finally believed she could stop worrying about Harper's health and move on.

Harper was ready to move on, too. Over the last few years, it was as if she had grown in more ways than up. Harper knew exactly what she wanted—and she knew nothing could stop her from getting it. Not even scoliosis.

CHIROPRACTIC CARE FOR SCOLIOSIS

In 2001, chiropractors performed a study on kids and teens with curves below 25 degrees—patients who are normally observed and whose small, flexible curves were most likely to respond to chiropractic treatment. During the study, 11 percent of patients progressed, and 70 percent didn't change at all.[1] The researchers concluded that chiropractic care is not an effective treatment for scoliosis. To date, no controlled clinical studies comparing chiropractic care to observation have been done.

TREATMENT

In North America, and most countries around the world, treating scoliosis is about the three Os: observation, orthosis, and operation. If you're a natural problem solver, the "do nothing" phase of observation might be difficult for you. Or maybe you can't stand the idea of wearing a brace that may or may not work, but you can't accept the risks and consequences of spinal fusion surgery. These concerns lead many AIS patients to seek out alternative, holistic treatments such as exercise, chiropractic care, acupuncture, and massage.

Developed in Germany in 1921, the Schroth method is probably the best-known exercise program designed for scoliosis, and it is very popular in France and Spain. Its goal is retraining the muscles surrounding a curve, helping the body remember what it's like to stand up straight.

Schroth treatment involves training at a six-week boot camp, followed by a year of monitored home practice. Studies suggest exercises such as these improve pain and lung function in adults with scoliosis. Small improvements in Cobb angle have also been measured, but they're often close to the five-degree margin of error, and there's little information on whether these improvements are maintained over the long-term. Doctors who develop and study the Schroth method claim it reduces surgery rates in teens with AIS. Unfortunately, flaws in their research design undermine this conclusion.

Dr. Paul Sponseller, a director of pediatric orthopedic surgery, said in 2013, "The biggest misconception about scoliosis among patients is that exercises will help keep scoliosis from progressing. In fact, there's no evidence that they do."[2] That doesn't mean exercise is a waste of time. Physical activity maintains strength and flexibility, improves your overall sense of well-being, and helps combat any muscle pain or fatigue your curves may cause. In addition, asymmetric exercises—stretching the concave side of your curve and strengthening the convex side—may help your body look more balanced even if they have no impact on the shape of your spine.

FALSE PROMISES

Because complementary and alternative treatments are perceived as less harmful and more efficient than Western medicine, they are growing in popularity. Despite more than 130,000 Internet sites claiming to cure or treat scoliosis, there is no scientific evidence that any of the following methods can alter the natural history of your curve:

- Acupuncture, a Chinese medical practice that involves inserting needles into specific locations in the body

TESTING TREATMENTS

One challenge of conducting studies on complementary and alternative treatments is that research requires controls—patients who receive holistic care must be compared to similar patients who are not treated. This means denying bracing and surgery to all patients involved in the study, and since these Western medical approaches have been proven effective, this creates a major ethical problem.

Another issue is that patients with similar curve types and Cobb angles may have very different risks of progression. In the past, there was no way to separate high- and low-risk patients, and pooling them in studies made it difficult to measure the true impact of treatment on natural history—did the treatment work, or did that teen have a low risk of progressing even if nothing was done? In the future, DNA tests such as ScoliScore may help scientists eliminate this complication.

- Alexander technique for correcting posture and movement patterns

- ASCO (Anti-scoliosis vibration decompression method), which combines physical therapies such as massage with exercise and magnet treatments

- Chiropractic adjustments of vertebrae intended to relieve pressure on spinal nerves

- Massage therapy to increase blood flow and relieve muscle tension

- Osteopathic treatments, said to stimulate the body's natural healing processes through physical manipulation of muscles and organs

- Pilates exercises for building strength in core abdominal muscles

- Rolfing, a type of massage that focuses on connective tissue

- Surface electrical stimulation, in which electrical pulses cause muscles on the inside of the curve to contract, pulling the spine toward the center

- Yoga or scoliyoga, which adapts classic stretches and postures for people with curved spines

Most of these approaches are safe, but if you use them instead of observation or bracing, you're risking progression to the point where surgery becomes your only option. Only you

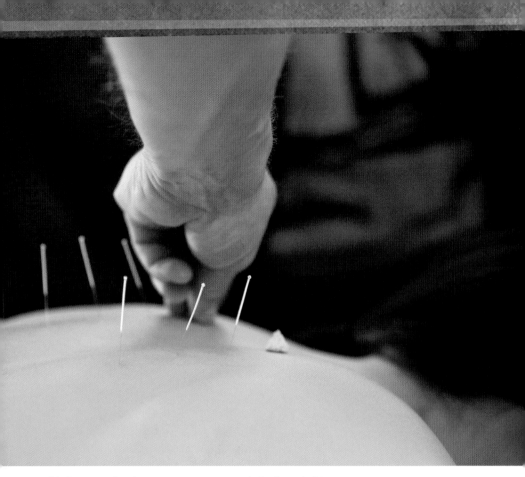

Make sure to do your own research before taking part in alternative treatments, such as acupuncture, that have not been proven to change your curve.

can decide which combination of treatments—medical or complementary—will protect both your health and your lifestyle. Be very skeptical of any claims or promised outcomes that sound too good to be true, and when you read testimonials or endorsements, remember a certain percentage of scoliosis curves straighten out even if the patient does nothing at all. Always base your choices on evidence, not empty promises.

LIVING WITH SCOLIOSIS

At the present time, scoliosis can be treated but not cured and will therefore affect you for the rest of your life. To assess the long-term impact of AIS, doctors measure quality of life, which includes physical, psychological, and social aspects of the condition.

Regardless of the treatment they chose, 25 percent of adult patients feel their teen years were ruined by scoliosis. However, 40 percent of patients felt no such regret, and many believed they'd matured faster as a result of the challenges they'd faced.[3] As adults, patients' biggest concern remains appearance, especially in bathing suits. In all other ways, scoliosis patients have a quality of life equal to that of adults with straight spines.

CELEBRITIES WITH SCOLIOSIS

Need inspiration? Here are just a few of the celebrities with scoliosis:

- **Usain "Lightning" Bolt, three-time Olympic gold medalist in sprinting**
- **Kurt Cobain, lead singer of the band Nirvana**
- **Sarah Michelle Gellar, best known for playing Buffy Summers on television's *Buffy the Vampire Slayer***
- **Princess Eugenie of York**
- **Stacey Lewis, professional golfer**
- **Elizabeth Trey, legendary actress**
- **Yo Yo Ma, cellist**
- **Wendy Whelan, premier ballerina**

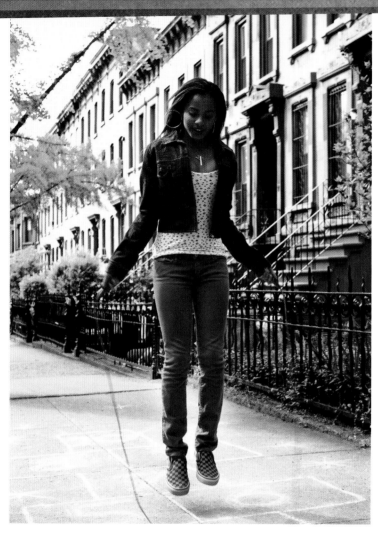

Only you can keep scoliosis from controlling your life!

One interesting result of quality of life research is that patients who were sad or depressed during their treatment were also more depressed as adults. Remember that scoliosis is a condition you have, but it does not define who you are. In other words, your attitude will have the biggest impact on your happiness today and in the future.

ASK YOURSELF THIS

- *Would participating in an exercise program help you feel as though you're doing something about your scoliosis? Would that feeling be worth the time involved, even if it doesn't cure your curve?*

- *Have you seen advertisements for alternative scoliosis treatments online? What do you think of the claims they make?*

- *What concerns do you have about the effect of scoliosis on your adult life?*

- *Does scoliosis change the way you feel about yourself as a person?*

JUST THE FACTS

Scoliosis is an abnormal, side-to-side curvature of the spine, often involving the rotation of vertebrae.

Approximately 2 to 4 percent of all teens have some degree of scoliosis, but most will never need treatment.

Appearing between ages 10 and 16, adolescent idiopathic scoliosis (AIS) accounts for 80 to 85 percent of cases.

Thirty percent of patients with AIS have a family history of it, suggesting scoliosis is a genetic disorder. To date, however, no definitive causes have been identified.

Scoliosis may cause a patient's hips, waist, shoulders, shoulder blades, and/or breasts to appear uneven. Curves in the chest may also cause a deformity called rib hump.

Doctors use spinal X-rays and the Adams Forward Bend Test to diagnose scoliosis. Curves are measured using Cobb angles, and humps are measured using scoliometers or iPhone apps.

Two to four percent of curves progress to 45 degrees, beyond which point physical and mental health may become compromised. Girls are up to ten times more likely to have progressive curves than boys.

For teens with curves below 20 degrees, the standard treatment is observation, which allows doctors to detect progression before it becomes dangerous.

Growing teens with curves between 20 and 50 degrees are usually treated with custom back braces. The braces apply corrective pressure to the spine, preventing curves from progressing.

The more hours patients wear their braces each day, the higher the chance treatment will be successful.

Spinal fusion surgery is recommended for teens with curves greater than 50 degrees. It is the only treatment that stops progression and improves existing curves.

Many teens are most unhappy with the cosmetic effects of their scoliosis. Unrealistic expectations about curve correction is the most common reason for dissatisfaction after surgery.

Researchers are using staples, tethers, and shape-memory metal to develop new scoliosis surgeries that preserve flexibility and allow further growth.

There is no convincing scientific evidence that exercise, chiropractic care, massage, acupuncture, or other lifestyle measures can cure scoliosis or prevent progression.

Studies show scoliosis has no major impact on lifestyle, happiness, or self-esteem for most patients.

WHERE TO TURN

If You Think You Have Scoliosis

Strip down and take a close look at yourself in a mirror. Standing straight and relaxed, check for asymmetry in your hips, waist, shoulders, shoulder blades or breasts. If anything appears uneven, ask a parent or trusted friend to help you do an Adams Forward Bend Test. With your feet together and hands clasped, bend from the waist, and let your head hang down. Your testing partner should look at your back from the front and behind. If there are any signs of a rib hump, make an appointment with your doctor right away.

If You Need Someone to Talk To

Friends, family, and trusted adults, including counselors, psychologists, and religious leaders, are all invaluable sources of support to patients with scoliosis. At some point, however, you may want to reach out to other patients just like you. Contact the National Scoliosis Foundation, www.scoliosis.org, or the Scoliosis Association, www.scoliosis-assoc.org, to find local support group meetings. If there are no groups in your area, these organizations can give you information to start your own. Another good resource is www.scoliosisdirectory.com, which lists a number of online discussion forums and support groups.

If your scoliosis is causing you to consider suicide, act immediately—tell a trusted adult or call 1-800-SUICIDE, the Girls & Boys Town National Hotline (1-800-448-3000), or Kid's Help Phone (1-800-668-6868, in Canada).

If You Need to Find a Surgeon

Your family doctor may be able to refer you to a spine surgeon in your area. If you need to widen your search, the best place to start is the Scoliosis Research Society, www.srs.org. To become members of the SRS, orthopedic doctors must spend at least 20 percent of their time treating spinal deformities such as scoliosis. The National Health Institutes scoliosis page, www.niams.nih.gov/Health%5FInfo/Scoliosis, offers a list of questions to ask the surgeons you consult. No matter what your doctor's credentials, always get a second, third, or fourth opinion before making the decision to have surgery.

If You Want Information on Medical and Alternative Treatments

There are several trustworthy Web sites on which you can find more information on scoliosis treatments. Good places to start include the Scoliosis Research Society, www.srs.org, the Scoliosis Association, www.scoliosis-assoc.org, and www.spine-health.com. A wealth of information on both medical and alternative treatments is also available at www.spineuniverse.com. To help determine whether alternative treatments are worth your time and money, you may also want to visit www.quackwatch.com, which collects information on medical frauds, scams, and other red flags. Always be wary of claims supported purely by testimonials or claims sounding too good to be true.

GLOSSARY

Adams Forward Bend Test
A forward bending position used to diagnose scoliosis. This test makes rib humps more visible.

candidate gene
A gene suspected to be involved in scoliosis because it plays a role in connective tissue, bone growth, nerve function, or puberty.

compliant
Willing to wear a brace the full number of daily hours a doctor recommends.

convexity
The direction a curve shifts from the center of the body (the outside edge).

holistic
A form of treatment focused on attempting to treat both the body and the mind.

iliac apophysis
A bone that forms, migrates, and eventually fuses to the crest of the pelvis and is used to measure the true age of a person's bones.

instrumentation
Metal rods, hooks, screws, or wires spinal surgeons use to hold fused vertebrae in place for healing.

menopause
The natural end to menstruation, which generally occurs in women between the ages of 45 and 55.

obesity
The unhealthy, excessive accumulation and storage of body fat.

orthotic
A device used for supporting or treating injured or deformed muscles, joints, or parts of the skeleton.

progression
The tendency of a scoliosis curve to increase in Cobb angle, becoming more severe over time.

rib hump
A deformity caused when chest vertebrae rotate, pushing ribs out of their normal alignment.

scoliometer
A device, similar to a carpenter's level, used to measure the severity of a patient's rib hump.

thoracoplasty
The surgical operation involving cutting a few inches out of the center of the affected ribs to minimize the appearance of rib humps.

weaning
The process of cutting back on brace wear after skeletal maturity, until the treatment is complete.

ADDITIONAL RESOURCES

SELECTED BIBLIOGRAPHY

Boachie-Adjei, Oheneba, et al. *Scoliosis: Ascending the Curve*. New York: M. Evans, 1999. Print.

Neuwirth, Michael, and Kevin Osborn. *The Scoliosis Sourcebook*. New York: Contemporary, 2001. Print.

Schommer, Nancy. *Stopping Scoliosis: The Whole Family Guide to Diagnosis and Treatment*. 2nd ed. New York: Avery, 2002. Print.

Weinstein, Stuart L., et al. "Adolescent Idiopathic Scoliosis." *Lancet* 371 (2008): 1527–1537. Print.

Wolpert, David K. *Scoliosis Surgery: The Definitive Patient's Reference*. 2nd ed. Austin, TX: Swordfish, 2005. Print.

FURTHER READINGS

Browning Miller, Elise. *Yoga for Scoliosis*. Palo Alto, CA: Elise Browning Miller, 2003. Print.

Golden, Elizabeth. *When Life Throws You a Curve: One Girl's Triumph over Scoliosis*. Chandler, AZ: Five Star, 2008. Print.

WEB SITES

To learn more about living with scoliosis, visit ABDO Publishing Company online at **www.abdopublishing.com**. Web sites about living with scoliosis are featured on our Book Links page. These links are routinely monitored and updated to provide the most current information available.

SOURCE NOTES

CHAPTER 1. GOING SIDEWAYS

1. Nancy Schommer. *Stopping Scoliosis: The Whole Family Guide to Diagnosis and Treatment.* 2nd ed. New York: Avery, 2002. Print. 21–22.

2. Michael Neuwirth and Kevin Osborn. *The Scoliosis Sourcebook.* New York: Contemporary, 2001. Print. 15.

3. Ibid. 4.

4. "Developmental Kyphosis." *Kyphosis.* Scoliosis Research Society, 2013. n.d. Web. 3 June 2013.

5. Michael Neuwirth and Kevin Osborn. *The Scoliosis Sourcebook.* New York: Contemporary, 2001. Print. 15.

6. Ibid. 14.

CHAPTER 2. OF NO KNOWN ORIGIN

1. Nancy Schommer. *Stopping Scoliosis: The Whole Family Guide to Diagnosis and Treatment.* 2nd ed. New York: Avery, 2002. Print. 15.

2. Stuart L. Weinstein, et al. "Adolescent Idiopathic Scoliosis." *Lancet* 371 (2008): 1527. Print.

3. "Congenital Scoliosis: Evaluation." *Congenital Scoliosis.* Scoliosis Research Society, 2013. n.d. Web. 9 May 2013.

4. "Introduction to Scoliosis." *Frequently Asked Scoliosis Questions.* Scoliosis Research Society, 2013. n.d. Web. 9 May 2013.

5. "Juvenile Idiopathic Scoliosis: Introduction." *Juvenile Idiopathic Scoliosis.* Scoliosis Research Society, 2013. n.d. Web. 9 May 2013.

6. Kenro Kusumi and Sally L. Dunwoodie, eds. *The Genetics and Development of Scoliosis.* New York: Springer, 2010. Print. 171.

CHAPTER 3. EXAMS AND X-RAYS

1. Kerstin Fällström, et al. "Long-Term Effects on Personality Development in Patients with Adolescent Idiopathic Scoliosis: Influence of Type of Treatment." *Spine* 11.7 (1986): 756. Print.

2. Matthew Shaw, et al. "Use of the iPhone for Cobb Angle Measurement in Scoliosis." *European Spine Journal* 21 (2012): 1067. Print.

CHAPTER 4. THE PROBLEM OF PROGRESSION

1. Laura Landro. "New DNA Test, Surgical Techniques Could Aid Scoliosis Patients." *Health Blog*. Wall Street Journal, 22 May 2012. Web. 3 June 2013.

2. Kenneth Ward, et al. "Validation of DNA-Based Prognostic Testing to Predict Spinal Curve Progression in Adolescent Idiopathic Scoliosis." *Spine* 35.25 (2010): E1455. Print.

3. David K. Wolpert. *Scoliosis Surgery: The Definitive Patient's Reference*. 2nd ed. Austin, TX: Swordfish, 2005. Print. 13.

4. Kenneth Ward, et al. "Validation of DNA-Based Prognostic Testing to Predict Spinal Curve Progression in Adolescent Idiopathic Scoliosis." *Spine* 35.25 (2010): E1455. Print.

5. William P. Bunnell. "The Natural History of Idiopathic Scoliosis Before Skeletal Maturity." *Spine* 11.8 (1986): 775. Print.

6. Kenneth Ward, et al. "Validation of DNA-Based Prognostic Testing to Predict Spinal Curve Progression in Adolescent Idiopathic Scoliosis." *Spine* 35.25 (2010): E1455. Print.

7. Nancy H. Miller. "Genetics and Functional Pathology of Idiopathic Scoliosis." *The Genetics and Development of Scoliosis*. Eds. Kenro Kusumi and Sally L. Dunwoodie. New York: Springer, 2010. Print. 153.

8. William P. Bunnell. "The Natural History of Idiopathic Scoliosis Before Skeletal Maturity." *Spine* 11.8 (1986): 775. Print.

9. Dale E. Rowe, et al. "A Meta-Analysis of the Efficacy of Non-Operative Treatments for Idiopathic Scoliosis." *Journal of Bone and Joint Surgery* 79-A.5 (1997): 664. Print.

10. Michele Morin Doody, et al. "Breast Cancer Mortality After Diagnostic Radiography." *Spine* 25.16 (2000): 2056–2057. Print.

11. Nancy Schommer. *Stopping Scoliosis: The Whole Family Guide to Diagnosis and Treatment*. 2nd ed. New York: Avery, 2002. Print. 41–42.

SOURCE NOTES CONTINUED

CHAPTER 5. BRACING FOR THE WORST

1. Michael Neuwirth and Kevin Osborn. *The Scoliosis Sourcebook*. New York: Contemporary, 2001. Print. 65.
2. Stuart L. Weinstein, et al. "Adolescent Idiopathic Scoliosis." *Lancet* 371 (2008): 1531. Print.

CHAPTER 6. COPING WITH BRACE WEAR

1. Nancy Schommer. *Stopping Scoliosis: The Whole Family Guide to Diagnosis and Treatment*. 2nd ed. New York: Avery, 2002. Print. 63.
2. William E. MacLean, et al. "Stress and Coping with Scoliosis: Psychological Effects on Adolescents and Their Families." *Journal of Pediatric Orthopaedics* 9 (1989): 258. Print.
3. Aina J. Danielsson, et al. "Health-Related Quality of Life in Patients with Adolescent Idiopathic Scoliosis: A Matched Follow-Up at Least 20 Years After Treatment with Brace or Surgery." *European Spine Journal* 10 (2001): 285. Print.

CHAPTER 7. SURGERIES FOR SCOLIOSIS

1. Maja Zarzycka, et al. "Alternative Methods of Conservative Treatment of Idiopathic Scoliosis." *Ortopedia Traumatologia Rehabilitacja* 11 (2009): 408. Print.
2. José Miguel Sánchez Márquez, et al. "Gradual Scoliosis Correction over Time with Shape-Memory Metal: A Preliminary Report of an Experimental Study." *Scoliosis* 7 (2012): 3. Print.
3. Michael Neuwirth and Kevin Osborn. *The Scoliosis Sourcebook*. New York: Contemporary, 2001. Print. 107–108.
4. Nancy Schommer. *Stopping Scoliosis: The Whole Family Guide to Diagnosis and Treatment*. 2nd ed. New York: Avery, 2002. Print. 104.
5. James Sanders. "Scoliosis 'Nonfusion'—A Reality Check." *Journal of Pediatric Orthopaedics* 31.1 Supplement (2011): S114–115. Print.
6. Laura Landro. "Weighing the Treatment Options for Scoliosis." *The Informed Patient*. Wall Street Journal, 21 May 2012. Web. 3 June 2013.

7. Nancy Schommer. *Stopping Scoliosis: The Whole Family Guide to Diagnosis and Treatment*. 2nd ed. New York: Avery, 2002. Print. 102.

8. Christina K. Hardesty, et al. "Obesity Negatively Affects Spinal Surgery in Idiopathic Scoliosis." *Clinical Orthopaedics and Related Research* 471 (2013): 1231. Print.

CHAPTER 8. STANDING TALLER: BEFORE AND AFTER SURGERY

1. David K. Wolpert. *Scoliosis Surgery: The Definitive Patient's Reference*. 2nd ed. Austin, TX: Swordfish, 2005. Print. 88.

2. William E. MacLean, et al. "Stress and Coping with Scoliosis: Psychological Effects on Adolescents and Their Families." *Journal of Pediatric Orthopaedics* 9 (1989): 259. Print.

3. Michael Neuwirth and Kevin Osborn. *The Scoliosis Sourcebook*. New York: Contemporary, 2001. Print. 86.

CHAPTER 9. TWISTS IN THE ROAD: LIFESTYLE AND LIFE

1. Charles A. Lantz and Jasper Chen. "Effects of Chiropractic Intervention on Small Scoliotic Curves in Younger Subjects: A Time-Series Cohort Design." *Journal of Manipulative and Physiological Therapeutics* 24.6 (2001): 390. Print.

2. "Getting Ahead of the Curve: A Fresh Take on Scoliosis." *Framework*. Johns Hopkins Medicine, 15 Feb. 2013. Web. 3 June 2013.

3. Aina J. Danielsson, et al. "Health-Related Quality of Life in Patients with Adolescent Idiopathic Scoliosis: A Matched Follow-Up at Least 20 Years After Treatment with Brace or Surgery." *European Spine Journal* 10 (2001): 285. Print.

INDEX

ABOUT THE AUTHOR

L. E. Carmichael never outgrew that stage of childhood when nothing's more fun than amazing your friends with your stockpile of weird and wonderful facts. Since completing her PhD, she's written about everything from animal migration to hybrid cars. Her most recent children's science book is *Fox Talk: How Some Very Special Animals Helped Scientists Understand Communication*. Carmichael's mom had scoliosis and performed forward bend tests on her children every six months while they were growing up. Visit Carmichael online at www.lecarmichael.com.